PREGNANCY GUIDE

Practical and Essential Tips for Every Expecting Mother

Introduction

Pregnancy Guide: Practical and Essential Tips for Every Expecting Mother

In the tapestry of life, there exists a chapter that is unlike any other a chapter woven with the threads of anticipation, wonder, and the profound magic of creation. This chapter, resplendent with the hues of love and vulnerability, unfolds in the sacred space where a woman nurtures life within her very being. Welcome to the realm of pregnancy a journey that is both universal and uniquely personal, a journey of transformation, discovery, and the profoundest of connections.

The creation of life is a miracle that transcends the boundaries of time, cultures, and languages. It is a universal experience that unites women across continents and generations. The journey from the moment of conception to the first cry of a newborn spans the spectrum of human emotions, from joy and excitement to apprehension and introspection. It is a journey that reshapes lives, redefines identities, and brings forth a love that knows no bounds.

In this monumental journey, guidance is invaluable. As with any grand expedition, traversing the landscapes of pregnancy necessitates maps, tools, and a compass. This guide, "Pregnancy Guide: Practical and Essential Tips for Every Expecting Mother," is designed to be that guiding light, that trusty companion that walks alongside you through the seasons of pregnancy. This is not just a book; it is a lantern that illuminates the path, a shelter that offers solace, and a treasure chest of wisdom that empowers you to navigate the unknown with confidence and grace.

The Journey of Motherhood

The journey of motherhood begins long before the first kick, the initial ultrasound, or even the momentous positive pregnancy test. It begins in the whispers of dreams, in the hopes woven through generations, and in the aspirations that rise from the deepest corners of the heart. This journey is more than a physical one; it is an emotional, spiritual, and psychological odyssey that stretches beyond the horizon of our understanding.

From the very instant of conception, when two cells fuse to form a new life, the symphony of existence takes on a new rhythm. The heartbeats synchronize, the blood flows in harmony, and the promise of a new dawn begins to unfurl. This transformation is not only about the body adapting to accommodate life; it is about the soul evolving, about the layers of one's identity deepening, and about the emotional tides that ebb and flow.

The journey of pregnancy is akin to writing an unwritten story. Each kick, each craving, and each moment of reflection contributes to a narrative that is uniquely yours. It is a story of resilience, of strength unearthed from the deepest wellsprings, and of the miracles that unfold within and around you. It is an

honor and a privilege to become a vessel of life, a guardian of dreams, and a conduit of love.

The Art of Nurturing

Nurturing is an art one that requires tenderness, attention, and a deep understanding of the subject. As you embark on the journey of pregnancy, you step into the role of a nurturer, both for yourself and for the life blossoming within. This art is not limited to the physical; it extends to the emotional, intellectual, and even spiritual dimensions of existence.

Nurturing oneself during pregnancy is not a luxury; it is a necessity. The physical changes are evident, but the emotional shifts are equally profound. Pregnancy is a time of rediscovering the self, of examining beliefs, and of forging a new relationship with the body. It is a time to listen to the whispers of intuition, to honor the body's needs, and to cocoon the spirit in an atmosphere of love and understanding.

But nurturing also involves acquiring knowledge

knowledge that empowers you to make informed choices, knowledge that dispels myths, and knowledge that equips you with the tools to embark on this journey with confidence. This guide aims to be your wellspring of knowledge, offering insights into the science, the emotions, and the complexities that intertwine during pregnancy.

Empowerment: The Beacon of Light

Empowerment is more than a word; it is a beacon of light that guides you through the often uncharted waters of pregnancy. Empowerment is the realization that you have the authority to make choices that resonate with your values, that you have the capability to embrace change with resilience, and that you have the strength to honor the journey you are undertaking.

In a world that often bombards us with conflicting advice and information, empowerment acts as an anchor. It enables you to sift through the noise and focus on what truly matters. It gives you the tools to navigate the challenges and the uncertainties that may arise, transforming them into opportunities for growth and learning.

Empowerment is also the understanding that each woman's journey is unique. What works for one may not work for another. The journey is not about adhering to a predefined set of rules; it is about carving your own path and weaving your own narrative. Empowerment allows you to embrace your journey with authenticity, authenticity that is rooted in the truth of who you are and the dreams you hold.

The Symphony of Content

This guide is a symphony a symphony composed of different notes, each contributing to the resonance of the whole. The content is carefully curated to provide a holistic understanding of pregnancy, addressing physical, emotional, and practical aspects. It is a tapestry woven with practical advice, scientific insights, real-life stories, and reflective exercises.

The chapters that follow are an exploration of the trimesters the progression of pregnancy that unfolds in three acts. From the fluttering whispers of the first trimester to the crescendo of anticipation in the third, each trimester has its own tale to tell. It is a tale of body and soul, of heartbeats and dreams, of transformations and revelations.

A Call to Journey

As you hold this guide in your hands, you hold more than just pages and words. You hold a key that opens the door to a journey of self-discovery, empowerment, and connection. This guide is a call to journey, an invitation to explore the landscapes of pregnancy with curiosity and courage.

May these pages become a sanctuary for your

questions, a wellspring for your insights, and a companion for your reflections. May the wisdom within these pages be a guiding star, lighting your way as you traverse the uncharted territories of pregnancy. And may the journey you undertake be one of profound transformation, of boundless love, and of the empowerment that arises from knowing that you possess the strength to embrace every facet of this miraculous journey.

With a heart brimming with excitement, anticipation, and gratitude, let us embark on this voyage together.

CONTENT

Chapter 1:

Embarking on the Journey
of Motherhood

The Miracle of Pregnancy. Embracing the Transformation.

In the quiet corners of existence, where the echoes of ancient stories and the whispers of generations past converge, there is a moment of profound magic a moment when life takes its first breath within the cocoon of a woman's body. It is a moment that defies the boundaries of language and science, transcending the realms of the known into the vast expanse of wonder. This moment, this miracle, is the genesis of a journey that will transform not only a woman's body but her very essence. Welcome to the realm of pregnancy a journey that encapsulates the beauty of creation, the awe of transformation, and the profound connection that binds mothers throughout time and space.

The Miracle of Pregnancy: A Symphony of Cells

The journey of pregnancy begins with a whisper a whisper that originates at the intersection of two sets of DNA, two intricate blueprints of life. It is at this juncture, within the depths of the woman's body, that a symphony of cells orchestrates a process of division and multiplication, a process that will ultimately lead to the creation of a new life. This magical fusion of cells, a dance that has been choreographed since the dawn of existence, ignites the spark of life that will flicker and burn brightly over the course of nine months.

The miracle of pregnancy is not solely about the scientific mechanics of cell division; it is about the emotional crescendo that accompanies it. From the moment of conception, a narrative unfolds a narrative that is woven with dreams, hopes, and the whispers of generations that have come before. It is a narrative that speaks of the continuation of life, of the endurance of humanity, and of the boundless love that brings new beings into the world.

Within the secret chambers of the womb, the dance of creation is guided by unseen hands. It is a dance of

delicate balance, a symphony of codes written in the language of DNA. The embryo begins to take shape, a minuscule vessel of potential, as the heart starts its rhythm, echoing the promise of a heartbeat that will echo throughout a lifetime. It is in these earliest moments that the foundation is laid a foundation upon which the entire journey of motherhood will be built.

Embracing the Transformation: A Journey of Becoming

As the embryo evolves into a fetus, a transformation of epic proportions unfolds within the woman's body. This transformation is not solely a physical one; it is an intricate tapestry woven from threads of change that extend beyond the boundaries of flesh and bone. It is a journey of becoming a journey that heralds the arrival of a new identity, that of a mother.

The transformation begins as the body adapts to the influx of hormones, the surge of growth, and the ebb and flow of emotions. The belly swells, signaling the growth of the tiny life nestled within. It is a miraculous spectacle the physical embodiment of the journey that has taken root within. Every inch gained by the belly is a testament to the marvel of existence, a reminder that life is unfolding in its purest form.

Yet, the transformation extends beyond the visible. It is the realization that the heart has expanded to accommodate a love that knows no bounds. It is the stirring of emotions—emotions that surge and recede like the tides, emotions that carry the weight of anticipation, excitement, and, at times, apprehension. It is the redefinition of priorities, the reshuffling of desires, and the surrender to a journey that transcends the individual and becomes a legacy.

Embracing the transformation is about surrendering to the unknown, about relinquishing control and allowing the currents of life to carry you forward. It is about acknowledging that this journey is not linear, that it is a tapestry woven with both triumphs and trials. It is about finding beauty in vulnerability, strength in surrender, and empowerment in the recognition that every stretch mark, every ache, and every emotional fluctuation is a brushstroke in the masterpiece of motherhood.

Bridging Time and Space: A Connection Through Generations

Pregnancy is a journey that bridges time and space a journey that connects women across continents, cultures, and epochs. As you embark on this transformative voyage, you become a part of a lineage that extends back to the earliest days of humanity. You walk in the footsteps of mothers who have cradled life within them, who have marveled at the mysteries of existence, and who have nurtured dreams that have rippled through the fabric of time.

As you navigate the exhilarating highs and the poignant lows of pregnancy, remember that you are not alone. You are connected to a tapestry of women who have walked this path before you, who have felt the same fluttering of life within their wombs, and who have experienced the same waves of love, hope, and anticipation. This connection is a lifelin that offers solace, wisdom, and the assurance that you are part of a sacred sisterhood that transcends generations.

In the chapters that follow, we will delve deeper into the intricacies of pregnancy the physical changes, the emotional landscape, and the practical aspects that shape this extraordinary journey. We will unravel the science, explore the emotions, and offer practical guidance that will accompany you through each trimester, each milestone, and each revelation. Together, we will navigate the uncharted waters of motherhood, armed with knowledge, compassion, and the unwavering belief in the power of creation.

As you continue on this remarkable journey, may you find strength in the miracle of life, solace in the embrace of transformation, and the profound connection that unites mothers throughout time. Your journey is a chapter in the grand tapestry of existence a chapter that is uniquely yours yet intertwined with the stories of countless women who have embarked on this sacred pilgrimage before you.

With a heart full of wonder and anticipation, let us embrace the journey that lies ahead.

Chapter 2

Understanding the Science of Pregnancy

sacred pilgrimage before you.

With a heart full of wonder and anticipation, let us embrace the journey that lies ahead.

Chapter 2

Understanding the Science of Pregnancy

The Biology of Conception. Unraveling the Trimesters.

In the intricate tapestry of life, there exists a chapter of unparalleled complexity a chapter that begins with the union of cells so small that they are invisible to the naked eye. This chapter, shrouded in wonder and steeped in science, is the story of conception, gestation, and the miraculous journey of pregnancy. Welcome to the realm of understanding the science of pregnancy a journey that unveils the biological symphony behind the creation of life and the transformation of a woman's body.

The Biology of Conception: The Dance of Life

At the heart of every human being lies a story that begins with the merging of two sets of DNA a microscopic pas de deux that initiates the choreography of life. This dance, orchestrated by the laws of genetics and biology, marks the beginning of a journey that will forever alter the fabric of existence.

Conception, the spark that ignites the journey of pregnancy, is the result of a myriad of intricate processes that unfold within the depths of the female reproductive system.

The stage for this dance is set in the ovaries, where thousands of potential life carriers ovarian follicles lie in wait. With the onset of menstruation, these follicles are triggered to mature, releasing an egg that embarks on a journey down the fallopian tube. It is in this tube, amidst the delicate tendrils and the embrace of secreted fluids, that the magic of conception occurs.

Conception is the result of a chance encounter a delicate ballet between the released egg and the awaiting sperm. As the sperm journey through the female reproductive tract, guided by the intricate chemistry of hormones, only a select few manage to reach the egg. The fusion of these two cells is a symphony of genetics a blending of traits that have been passed down through generations, a merging of potentialities that will shape the unique individual that is being formed.

As these cells unite, they give rise to a zygote a single cell that holds the promise of life. This zygote, guided by the biological map encoded in its DNA, undergoes a series of divisions that result in the formation of a blastocyst. This blastocyst, brimming with potential, finds its way to the lining of the uterus, where it burrows in and establishes a connection with the mother's body a connection that will nurture and sustain the growing life.

Unraveling the Trimesters: A Journey of Development

As the blastocyst nestles within the uterine lining, the journey of pregnancy unfolds a journey marked by distinct stages known as trimesters. Each trimester is a chapter of development, a period of growth and transformation that is both awe-inspiring and carefully orchestrated by the intricate symphony of biology.

The First Trimester: A Prelude to Life

The first trimester is a time of incredible transformation a period marked by the inception of vital systems, the establishment of the placenta, and the onset of visible changes within the mother's body. As the blastocyst implants and the placenta begins to form, the body responds with the release of hormones that prevent the shedding of the uterine lining, thus sustaining the pregnancy.

During this period, the embryo goes through rapid changes. The neural tube forms, setting the foundation for the central nervous system, while the heart begins to beat, becoming the rhythm that will sustain life. The intricate dance of limb development, organogenesis, and cellular differentiation ensues, laying the groundwork for the intricate systems that will define the human body.

The Second Trimester: The Blossoming of Life

As the second trimester dawns, the embryo transitions into a fetus a transformation that heralds a period of rapid growth and blossoming. It is during this phase that the physical manifestations of pregnancy become more apparent the burgeoning belly, the fluttering movements, and the distinctive curve of life that has taken root.

The fetus undergoes remarkable development during the second trimester. The senses awaken as the eyes form, the ears take shape, and the sense of touch emerges. Reflexes develop, allowing for delicate movements, and the brain undergoes rapid growth, laying the foundation for cognitive and sensory capabilities.

The Third Trimester: A Prelude to Arrival

As the journey through the trimesters nears its culmination, the third trimester becomes a time of readiness a period when the fetus prepares for the journey from the womb into the world. The body matures in preparation for birth, with the lungs practicing breathing movements, the digestive system gearing up for nourishment, and the immune system receiving a boost from maternal antibodies.

The fetus's senses are finely tuned during the third trimester. It responds to external stimuli, recognizing sounds, voices, and even rhythms. The intricate dance of hormonal signals triggers contractions and readies the body for the intricate choreography of labor and delivery.

Bridging Science and Wonder: Embracing the Journey

Understanding the science of pregnancy is akin to unveiling the blueprint of creation—a blueprint that is rich with complexity, precision, and an orchestration that defies comprehension. The journey from conception to birth is a testament to the interplay of biology and nature, of genes and environments, and of the delicate balance that sustains life.

As you traverse the landscape of pregnancy, armed with the knowledge of biology, may you find solace in the scientific symphony that guides the journey. May the awareness of the remarkable processes unfolding within your body enhance the wonder and reverence you hold for the creation of life. From the fusion of cells to the formation of intricate organs, every step of this journey is a testimony to the brilliance of nature's design.

In the chapters that follow, we will delve deeper into the physical and emotional aspects of pregnancy, exploring the changes that unfold within the body and the heart. We will unravel the mysteries of prenatal care, offer insights into managing discomfort, and provide practical guidance to navigate the trimesters with confidence and grace.

As you continue on this remarkable journey, remember that you are part of an intricate biological tapestry a tapestry that has been woven since the dawn of existence. You are a steward of life, a guardian of transformation, and a bearer of the miracle that is pregnancy.

With a heart full of wonder and a mind enriched with knowledge, let us embrace the journey of understanding the science of pregnancy a journey that merges the realms of wonder and biology in a symphony of creation.

Chapter 3:

Nutrition for Two: Nourishing Your Body and Baby

Pregnancy Diet: What to Eat and Avoid. Essential Nutrients for a Healthy Pregnancy.

In the tapestry of life, nutrition is the thread that weaves through every stage a thread that takes on heightened significance during the transformative journey of pregnancy. Nourishing your body and your growing baby is not just a matter of sustenance; it is a profound act of love and responsibility. Welcome to the realm of nutrition for two a journey that explores the nuances of a pregnancy diet, unveils the essentials for a healthy pregnancy, and guides you toward making choices that nourish both you and your precious cargo.

Pregnancy Diet: What to Eat and Avoid

Within the realm of pregnancy, nutrition is more than just a collection of meals; it is a lifeline that fuels the growth of a new life, that sustains the well-being of the mother, and that creates a foundation for a healthy journey ahead. Crafting a pregnancy diet is a delicate art that involves making thoughtful choices, embracing balance, and nurturing your body as it undergoes remarkable changes.

Embracing Nutrient-Rich Foods

The cornerstone of a pregnancy diet lies in the embrace of nutrient-rich food that are abundant in vitamins, minerals, and essential macronutrients. Fruits and vegetables form the vibrant spectrum of colors that are not only visually appealing but also brimming with antioxidants, fiber, and vitamins. Whole grains provide a steady supply of energy, while lean proteins offer amino acids that support growth and development.

Omega-3 fatty acids, found in fatty fish, flaxseeds, and walnuts, are a precious addition to your pregnancy diet. These essential fats contribute to the development of your baby's brain and eyes, while also supporting your cardiovascular health.

Avoiding Harmful Substances

In the mosaic of pregnancy nutrition, avoidance is as important as embrace. Harmful substances, such as alcohol, tobacco, and certain types of fish high in mercury, should be avoided. Caffeine intake should be moderated, as excess caffeine can impact fetal development. Additionally, undercooked or raw foods should be approached with caution, as they carry the risk of foodborne illnesses.

Hydration: The Elixir of Life

Amidst the focus on solids, the role of hydration should never be underestimated. Water is the elixir of life essential for the circulation of nutrients, the removal of waste, and the maintenance of amniotic fluid levels. Staying well-hydrated supports overall well-being and can alleviate common discomforts such as constipation and edema.

Essential Nutrients for a Healthy Pregnancy

Within the framework of pregnancy nutrition lies a treasure trove of essential nutrients that play a pivotal role in nurturing the well-being of both the mother and the developing baby. These nutrients are the building blocks of life, the agents of growth, and the guardians of health.

Folate and Folic Acid: Guardian of Development

Folate, a B-vitamin, is a cornerstone of prenatal nutrition. Adequate folate intake, both before conception and during the early stages of pregnancy, is crucial for preventing neural tube defects. Folic acid, a synthetic form of folate, is often recommended as a supplement to ensure optimal intake.

Iron: Powering Oxygen Circulation

Iron is the mineral that powers oxygen transport throughout the body. During pregnancy, blood volume increases to accommodate the needs of both the mother and the growing baby. Adequate iron intake is vital to prevent anemia and support the formation of healthy red blood cells.

Calcium: Building Strong Bones and Teeth

Calcium is a mineral that is intricately tied to the formation of bones and teeth. It is of paramount importance during pregnancy, as the baby's skeletal development is underway. Ensuring adequate calcium intake is essential to prevent the mother's body from drawing upon her own bone stores to meet the growing baby's needs.

Vitamin D: The Sunshine Nutrient

Vitamin D, often referred to as the "sunshine vitamin," plays a crucial role in calcium absorption and bone health. This nutrient is particularly significant during pregnancy, as it supports the baby's skeletal development. Spending time in natural sunlight, consuming vitamin D-rich foods, or taking a supplement can help maintain optimal levels.

Protein: The Building Blocks of Life

Protein is the foundation upon which life is built. During pregnancy, protein is crucial for the growth of the placenta, the development of the baby's organs, and the maintenance of the mother's tissues. Lean meats, poultry, fish, eggs, dairy products, legumes, and nuts are excellent sources of protein.

Crafting a Balanced Pregnancy Diet

As you embark on the journey of nourishing your body and your baby, remember that balance is key. A balanced pregnancy diet includes a variety of nutrient-rich foods that offer an array of vitamins and minerals. The "eat a rainbow" philosophy encourages you to consume a diverse assortment of fruits and vegetables, each contributing its unique blend of nutrients to your diet.

Carbohydrates, often given an unfair reputation, are an essential source of energy. Opt for complex carbohydrates, such as whole grains, fruits, and vegetables, which provide sustained energy and fiber to support digestion.

Healthy fats, such as those found in avocados, nuts, seeds, and olive oil, are vital for the absorption of fat-soluble vitamins (A, D, E, and K) and contribute to the healthy development of your baby's brain.

Navigating Cravings and Aversions

Pregnancy is often accompanied by a rollercoaster of cravings and aversions a symphony of tastes and smells that can surprise even the most seasoned palate. While giving in to occasional cravings can be a source of comfort, it's important to maintain a balance and ensure that your nutritional needs are being met. If you find yourself craving specific foods, consider exploring healthier alternatives or incorporating those cravings into a well-rounded meal.

Likewise, aversions to certain foods are a common aspect of pregnancy. If a once-beloved dish no longer appeals to you, listen to your body and find alternative sources of the nutrients that food provided.

Cultivating Mindful Eating

Mindful eating is a practice that encourages you to engage with your meals in a way that promotes awareness, gratitude, and connection. During pregnancy, when the body is undergoing transformation, mindful eating becomes particularly relevant. Taking time to savor each bite, acknowledging the nourishment it offers, and being present in the act of eating can foster a deeper connection to both your body and your growing baby.

The Journey of Nourishment Continues

As you navigate the terrain of pregnancy nutrition, may you be inspired by the harmony that emerges when science and nourishment intertwine. The choices you make, the foods you embrace, and the care you bestow upon your body shape not only your well-being but also the development of a new life. Your journey of nourishment is a chapter of love, responsibility, and the profound connection that emerges when you nourish your body and your baby.

In the chapters that follow, we will delve deeper into the various aspects of pregnancy, exploring the physical changes, emotional landscape, and practical considerations that shape this extraordinary journey. We will unveil the art of self-care, offer guidance for coping with discomforts, and provide insights into embracing pregnancy with confidence and grace.

As you continue on this remarkable journey, may your nutrition choices reflect the reverence

you hold for the miracle of life. With a heart full of intention and a plate full of nourishment, let us embark on the voyage of nurturing your body and your growing baby a voyage that intertwines the threads of science, care, and love.

Chapter 4:

Physical Changes and Self-Care During Pregnancy

Body Changes: From Bumps to Swollen Feet. Pregnancy Fitness: Staying Active Safely.

In the grand tapestry of pregnancy, the body becomes a canvas of transformation a canvas painted with strokes of growth, change, and the remarkable journey of nurturing life. As your body adapts to the demands of pregnancy, it's a time not only for embracing these changes but also for nurturing yourself through self-care and mindful choices. Welcome to the realm of physical changes and self-care during pregnancy a journey that explores the intricacies of bodily transformation, offers insights into managing discomforts, and guides you in maintaining a healthy, active lifestyle.

Body Changes: From Bumps to Swollen Feet

Pregnancy is a time of metamorphosis—a time when the body, guided by the symphony of biology, transforms to accommodate the growing life within.

From the unmistakable bump that cradles your precious cargo to the subtle shifts that ripple through your skin, every physical change tells a story—a story of growth, adaptation, and the miracle of creation.

The Blossoming Bump

The most iconic and visible change during pregnancy is undoubtedly the blossoming bump. As your uterus expands to accommodate the growing baby, your abdomen takes on new contours a reflection of the life that is taking root within. Each day brings a subtle shift, an expansion that echoes the progress of pregnancy, and a canvas that carries the legacy of generations.

Skin Deep: Stretch Marks and Glow

As the body stretches to make room for the new life, the skin often reveals its own tale of transformation. Stretch marks, those silvery ribbons that weave across the abdomen, hips, and breasts, are a reminder of the incredible journey your body is undertaking. These marks, often referred to as "tiger stripes," tell a story of strength, growth, and the incredible resilience of the body.

The famed "pregnancy glow" is another hallmark of the physical changes during pregnancy. It's a radiant aura that envelops many expectant mothers a manifestation of increased blood flow, hormonal changes, and the joy that comes with nurturing life.

Swollen Feet and Beyond

As the months progress, the body's circulatory system undergoes changes that can lead to swelling, particularly in the feet and ankles. This swelling, known as edema, is often a result of the pressure exerted by the growing uterus on blood vessels. It serves as a gentle reminder of the intricate dance of biology and the temporary nature of these changes.

Managing these physical changes involves a blend of self-care, mindfulness, and acceptance. Embracing your evolving body with love and kindness is a powerful act one that honors the journey of pregnancy and the remarkable resilience of the human body.

Pregnancy Fitness: Staying Active Safely

Amidst the changes and challenges of pregnancy, the importance of staying active cannot be overstated. Engaging in safe and appropriate physical activity not only supports your physical well-being but also contributes to your emotional health and overall vitality.

The Benefits of Exercise

Exercise during pregnancy is not just about maintaining fitness; it's about optimizing your body's ability to support the demands of pregnancy and labor. Regular physical activity can alleviate common discomforts, enhance circulation, and even contribute to a smoother recovery postpartum. Additionally, exercise releases endorphins the "feel-good" hormones that can combat stress, anxiety, and mood fluctuations.

Safe and Suitable Activities

The journey to pregnancy fitness is marked by balance and mindfulness. While exercise is beneficial, it's crucial to choose activities that are safe and suitable for the changing needs of your body. Low-impact activities such as walking, swimming, stationary cycling, and prenatal yoga are excellent options that can be adapted to your fitness level and comfort.

Listen to your body's cues and communicate with your healthcare provider before starting or continuing an exercise regimen. It's important to be aware of any medical conditions or complications that might influence your exercise choices.

Pelvic Floor Health: A Vital Component

As you engage in physical activity during pregnancy, a special focus should be placed on pelvic floor health. The pelvic floor muscles, which support the bladder, uterus, and bowels, undergo significant changes during pregnancy and childbirth. Incorporating pelvic floor exercises, commonly known as Kegel exercises, can enhance your pelvic floor strength and reduce the risk of issues such as urinary incontinence.

Crafting a Self-Care Routine

Amidst the physical changes and the journey toward pregnancy fitness, self-care emerges as a guiding light a beacon of nurturing and mindfulness. Self-care during pregnancy is not a luxury; it's a necessity that supports your well-being and prepares you for the journey ahead.

Nurturing Body and Mind

Self-care takes many forms, from nurturing your body with nutrient-rich foods to embracing gentle movements that honor your physical well-being. It also involves fostering a deep connection between your mind and your body an awareness that allows you to listen to your body's cues and respond with compassion.

Rest and Rejuvenation

Rest becomes a form of self-care that is both vital and restorative. Pregnancy places demands on your body, and it's essential to grant yourself permission to rest when needed. Prioritize sleep, create moments of quiet contemplation, and explore relaxation techniques that promote inner calm.

Mindful Practices

Mindfulness is a powerful tool that can enhance your pregnancy journey. Engage in practices such as meditation, deep breathing, and gentle yoga to cultivate a sense of presence and peace. Mindful practices also facilitate a deeper connection to your growing baby, fostering a bond that extends beyond the physical.

Navigating the Journey with Confidence

The journey of physical changes and self-care during pregnancy is a testament to the incredible capabilities of the human body. As you embrace the metamorphosis that unfolds within, remember that you are participating in an age-old dance that generations of mothers have performed before you.

In the chapters that follow, we will delve deeper into the multifaceted landscape of pregnancy, exploring the emotional fluctuations, the preparations for childbirth, and the nurturing of your growing baby. We will unveil the art of emotional well-being, offer guidance for navigating labor and delivery, and provide insights into the incredible journey of motherhood.

As you continue on this remarkable journey, may you find solace in the embrace of self-care, marvel in the transformation of your body, and celebrate the strength that accompanies each physical change. Your journey is a symphony of growth, a dance of resilience, and a canvas upon which the masterpiece of pregnancy is painted.

With a heart full of reverence and a body full of wonder, let us navigate the terrain of physical changes and self-care a terrain that mirrors the grace and beauty of creation itself.

Chapter 5:

Nurturing Your Emotional Well-being

The Emotional Rollercoaster of Pregnancy. Mindfulness and Stress Relief.

In the intricate mosaic of pregnancy, emotions emerge as vibrant hues shades of joy, uncertainty, excitement, and vulnerability that paint the canvas of your experience. As your body undergoes transformation, so does your emotional landscape a terrain that deserves tender care and mindful attention. Welcome to the realm of nurturing your emotional well-being a journey that explores the emotional rollercoaster of pregnancy, offers insights into the art of mindfulness, and guides you toward strategies for stress relief and inner balance.

The Emotional Rollercoaster of Pregnancy

Pregnancy is a journey of heart and soul a journey that ushers in a wave of emotions, each as unique as a brushstroke on a canvas. From elation to anxiety, from wonder to worry, the emotional spectrum of pregnancy is rich and diverse, reflecting the profound changes unfolding within and around you.

The Symphony of Hormones

The emotional fluctuations of pregnancy are, in part, orchestrated by a symphony of hormones a complex composition that influences not only your body but also your mind. Hormones such as estrogen and progesterone surge and ebb, impacting neurotransmitters and triggering emotions that can be intense and unpredictable.

Mind and Body Connection

The connection between your emotional and physical states becomes evident during pregnancy. The changes in your body can sometimes amplify your emotions, leading to moments of heightened sensitivity, tears, or bursts of laughter. It's important to recognize that these emotional responses are valid and an intrinsic part of the journey.

Embracing the Spectrum

As you navigate the emotional rollercoaster of pregnancy, remember that each emotion is a valid part of the experience. From the sheer exhilaration of feeling your baby's first kick to the moments of doubt and worry, each emotion carries its own significance. Embrace this spectrum with an open heart, acknowledging that it is the tapestry of emotions that adds depth and richness to the journey.

Mindfulness and Stress Relief

Amidst the waves of emotions, mindfulness emerges as a lifeline an anchor that allows you to navigate the currents of pregnancy with grace and presence. Mindfulness is the practice of being fully present in the moment, cultivating awareness of your thoughts, feelings, and sensations without judgment. It's a powerful tool that can transform your emotional landscape and offer relief from stress and uncertainty.

The Art of Mindfulness

Mindfulness invites you to meet each moment with openness and curiosity a practice that can significantly impact your emotional well-being during pregnancy. Engaging in mindfulness exercises, such as meditation, deep breathing, and body scans, fosters a sense of centeredness and helps you manage the ebb and flow of emotions.

The Power of Presence

One of the gifts of mindfulness is the ability to shift your focus from past worries or future uncertainties to the present moment. When you cultivate mindfulness, you create a safe space within yourself a space where you can acknowledge your emotions without being overwhelmed by them. This presence allows you to respond to your emotions with compassion and self-care.

Mindful Self-Compassion

Self-compassion is a cornerstone of mindfulness a practice that involves treating yourself with the same kindness and understanding that you would offer to a dear friend. During pregnancy, when emotions can be particularly intense, self-compassion becomes an essential tool for nurturing your emotional well-being. When you're feeling overwhelmed or critical of yourself, imagine what you would say to a friend in the same situation, and offer those same words of comfort to yourself.

Strategies for Stress Relief

Stress, a common companion of modern life, can become amplified during pregnancy as you navigate both physical changes and emotional fluctuations. Incorporating strategies for stress relief is not only beneficial for your well-being but also supports the health of your growing baby.

Breathwork: A Gateway to Calm

Your breath is a constant companion a bridge that connects the inner landscape of your body with the external world. Breathwork, often integrated with mindfulness practices, is a potent tool for stress relief. Engage in deep, intentional breathing exercises that invite relaxation and a sense of inner calm.

Guided Imagery and Visualization

Guided imagery is a technique that harnesses the power of your imagination to create a mental retreat a safe haven of peace and tranquility. Through visualization, you can transport yourself to serene landscapes, immerse yourself in positive experiences, and ease your mind from stressors.

Connecting with Nature

Nature, with its soothing rhythms and gentle

whispers, offers a sanctuary for your emotional well-being. Take leisurely walks in a park, embrace the serenity of a beach, or find solace in the embrace of a forest. Connecting with nature not only reduces stress but also fosters a sense of connection to the larger world around you.

Crafting Inner Balance

Nurturing your emotional well-being is a journey of self-discovery a journey that encourages you to explore the nuances of your emotions, tend to your inner landscape, and embrace the beauty of imperfection. As you navigate the emotional terrain of pregnancy, remember that you possess the tools to cultivate inner balance and resilience.

Embracing Support

Seeking support during this journey is an act of strength and wisdom. Share your emotions with your partner, friends, family, or a mental health professional. Engaging in open conversations can alleviate feelings of isolation and provide perspectives that offer solace and understanding.

Honoring Your Needs

Your emotional well-being is interconnected with your physical, mental, and spiritual needs. Prioritize self-care, nourishing foods, rest, and activities that bring you joy. Engage in practices that uplift your spirits, such as creative expression, journaling, or engaging in hobbies you love.

The Journey of Emotion and Presence Continues

As you navigate the landscape of nurturing your emotional well-being, remember that your emotions are an integral part of the journey. Just as your body adapts to the physical changes of pregnancy, your heart and soul adapt to the emotional shifts with grace and resilience.

In the chapters that follow, we will delve deeper into the multifaceted landscape of pregnancy, exploring the preparation for childbirth, the art of bonding with your baby, and the transition into motherhood. We will unveil the practices that support a positive birth experience, offer guidance for early parenting, and provide insights into the profound journey of nurturing and raising a child.

As you continue on this remarkable journey, may you find solace in mindfulness, strength in embracing your emotions, and wisdom in nurturing your emotional well-being. Your journey is a testament to the beauty of the human experience a journey that weaves together the threads of body, heart, and soul.

With a heart full of presence and a spirit full of resilience, let us navigate the terrain of emotional well-being a terrain that reflects the intricate masterpiece of your inner world.

Chapter 6:

Building a Strong Support System

Partner, Family, and Friends: Navigating Relationships. Finding Your Pregnancy Tribe.

In the symphony of pregnancy, the power of connection emerges as a guiding theme a theme that underscores the importance of nurturing relationships, seeking support, and building a web of care around you. As you embark on the journey of motherhood, the foundation of a strong support system becomes an essential cornerstone. Welcome to the realm of building a strong support system a journey that explores the dynamics of partner, family, and friend relationships, and guides you in finding your pregnancy tribe a circle of understanding and camaraderie.

Partner, Family, and Friends: Navigating Relationships

Pregnancy is a transformative journey that ripples beyond the boundaries of your own experience, touching the lives of your partner, family, and friends. Navigating these relationships during this time requires sensitivity, communication, and a deep understanding of the shifting dynamics.

Partners in Parenthood

The journey of pregnancy is a shared voyage a voyage that both you and your partner embark upon together. As you anticipate the arrival of your baby, your partner's role becomes intertwined with the web of emotions, decisions, and experiences that shape this journey. Communication becomes a lifeline a channel through which you share your thoughts, fears, and hopes.

Honor the unique journey of your partner. While your experiences are deeply personal, your partner also navigates his or her own path of understanding and adaptation. Engage in open conversations, ask questions, and express your needs. Consider attending prenatal classes together, reading books on pregnancy and parenting, and discussing your birth plan. The journey of pregnancy is an opportunity to cultivate a deeper connection and a stronger bond as you anticipate the transformation of becoming parents.

Family Dynamics: A Tapestry of Perspectives

The journey of pregnancy often brings family dynamics to the forefront complex relationships that can be a source of joy, challenges, and a mosaic of perspectives. As you navigate interactions with extended family members, remember that each person brings their own experiences, beliefs, and expectations to the table.

Boundaries become an essential tool in maintaining your emotional well-being. Communicate your needs clearly and assertively, while also being open to understanding the perspectives of others. Surround yourself with individuals who uplift and support you, and consider seeking guidance from your healthcare provider or a mental health professional if family dynamics become particularly challenging.

Friends: The Tapestry of Camaraderie

Friendships are a source of light a tapestry of camaraderie that can be especially comforting during pregnancy. As you experience the changes and emotions that come with this journey, your friends can serve as pillars of support and understanding. They are often the ones who lend a listening ear, share in your joys and challenges, and offer words of encouragement.

Be selective in sharing your experiences with friends. Not everyone needs to be privy to the intimate details of your journey. Choose friends who are empathetic, respectful, and capable of providing the support you need. Communicate your boundaries and let them know how they can be there for you.

Finding Your Pregnancy Tribe

Amidst the journey of pregnancy, the concept of finding your pregnancy tribe emerges as a beacon of camaraderie and belonging. A pregnancy tribe consists of individuals who share in your experiences, who understand the nuances of the journey, and who offer unwavering support and companionship.

Online Communities and Forums

In the digital age, online communities and forums provide a virtual haven for expectant mothers seeking connection and advice. Joining platforms specifically tailored to pregnancy can introduce you to individuals who are navigating similar experiences. These communities can be valuable sources of information, as well as spaces to share your joys, concerns, and questions.

Prenatal Classes and Support Groups

Prenatal classes and support groups offer the opportunity to connect with individuals in person an avenue for forging meaningful relationships. Many communities offer classes on childbirth education, breastfeeding, and newborn care. Engaging in these classes not only provides you with valuable knowledge but also introduces you to fellow expectant parents who are on a similar journey.

Embracing Diversity

Your pregnancy tribe may include individuals from diverse backgrounds, experiences, and perspectives. Embrace the richness of these connections, as they can offer insights and wisdom that broaden your understanding of pregnancy and motherhood. The common thread that binds you is the shared journey of nurturing life, and this commonality can create strong bonds of friendship.

The Power of Support and Connection

Building a strong support system during pregnancy

is a profound act of self-care and self-compassion. Surrounding yourself with individuals who uplift you, understand your journey, and offer a listening ear can significantly impact your emotional well-being.

Effective Communication

Effective communication is the cornerstone of nurturing relationships during pregnancy. Express your needs, boundaries, and emotions clearly and openly. Encourage your partner, family, and friends to do the same. Healthy communication fosters understanding, minimizes misunderstandings, and strengthens the connections that support you.

Boundaries: A Shield of Self-Care

Setting boundaries is an act of self-preservation a shield that protects your emotional well-being. Be discerning in the information you share and the interactions you engage in. Politely assert your boundaries when needed, and prioritize your own comfort and needs.

The Journey of Connection and Care Continues

As you navigate the realm of building a strong support system, remember that connection is a lifeline a lifeline that nurtures your emotional well-being, offers solace in moments of doubt, and celebrates the joys of the journey. Your support system is a mosaic of relationships a tapestry that reflects the strength of human connection.

In the chapters that follow, we will delve deeper into the multifaceted landscape of pregnancy, exploring the preparations for childbirth, the art of bonding with your baby, and the transition into motherhood. We will unveil the practices that support a positive birth experience, offer guidance for early parenting, and provide insights into the incredible journey of nurturing and raising a child.

As you continue on this remarkable journey, may your support system offer a safe harbor, may your relationships be a source of strength, and may you find joy in building connections that uplift your spirit. Your journey is a symphony of camaraderie, a dance of connection, and a tapestry of care.

With a heart full of gratitude and a spirit full of connection, let us navigate the terrain of building a strong support system a terrain that echoes the beauty of human relationships.

Chapter 7:

Preparing Your Nest: The Practicalities of Baby Gear

Creating a Comfortable Living Space. The Essentials for Your Hospital Bag

As you journey through pregnancy, a symphony of anticipation unfolds the crescendo of excitement, preparation, and readiness for the arrival of your little one. Central to this preparation is the art of creating a nurturing living space and assembling the essentials for your hospital bag. Welcome to the realm of preparing your nest—a journey that explores the practicalities of setting up your home and packing for the hospital stay, ensuring that you're equipped with the tools and comforts needed for the momentous occasion ahead.

Creating a Comfortable Living Space

The space you inhabit becomes a sanctuary a cocoon that cradles the tender moments of pregnancy and the forthcoming adventure of parenthood. Creating a comfortable living space not only fosters a sense of calm but also ensures that you're well-prepared to welcome your baby into your home.

Nursery Nesting

Designing a nursery is a labor of love a canvas upon which you paint your dreams and aspirations for your baby. As you craft this space, remember that simplicity and functionality are your allies. Choose furniture that serves dual purposes, such as cribs that convert into toddler beds, and invest in ample storage solutions to keep baby essentials organized.

Consider the placement of the nursery in proximity to your own bedroom a practice that supports convenient nighttime feedings and check-ins. Opt for soft, neutral colors that create a serene atmosphere, and adorn the space with personalized touches that reflect your journey.

Baby Essentials: What You Truly Need

The world of baby gear is a vast landscape, filled with an array of gadgets and accessories. However, the key to creating a comfortable living space lies in discerning what you truly need. Prioritize essentials that cater to your baby's safety, comfort, and well-being.

A crib, a changing table, and a comfortable chair for feeding and cuddling are among the foundational pieces. Consider investing in a quality baby monitor to ensure your baby's safety even when you're not in the same room. Clothing, swaddle blankets, diapers, and feeding supplies are essential components that simplify the early days of parenthood.

The Essentials for Your Hospital Bag

The hospital bag is a tangible manifestation of your readiness a vessel that holds the essentials needed for your stay during childbirth and those precious first moments with your newborn. Packing thoughtfully ensures that you're equipped with both practical items and sentimental touches that offer comfort and familiarity.

For You: Comfort and Care

As you pack your hospital bag, prioritize comfort and care for yourself. Clothing that is loose, comfortable, and easy to change is essential for your stay. Consider pajamas, nursing bras, and maternity underwear. Toiletries, such as a toothbrush, toothpaste, and skincare products, offer a touch of normalcy during your hospital stay.

Pack snacks that provide nourishment and energy, as labor and delivery can be physically demanding. Additionally, include items that offer comfort and relaxation, such as a favorite pillow, soothing music, or a book.

For Baby: Welcoming Essentials

For your newborn, pack essentials that ensure a gentle and warm welcome. Baby clothing, onesies, and receiving blankets are among the must-haves. Consider including soft hats and mittens to protect your baby from drafts and prevent scratching. Diapers, wipes, and diaper cream are practical items that ensure your baby's comfort.

Pack a going-home outfit for your baby a special ensemble that marks the beginning of your journey as a family. Choose items that are weather-appropriate, considering both warmth and comfort.

The Tapestry of Preparation

The act of preparing your nest is more than just a checklist of items it's a tapestry woven with love, care, and anticipation. As you create a comfortable living space and pack your hospital bag, remember that these tangible preparations reflect your heart's readiness to welcome a new life into your home.

Organization and Preparation

Effective organization plays a crucial role in the

practicalities of preparing your nest. Create lists that outline the essentials for your nursery, ensuring that you prioritize safety and functionality. Similarly, compile a detailed list of items for your hospital bag, categorizing items for yourself, your partner, and your baby.

Personal Touches: An Intimate Thread

Amidst the practicalities, don't forget to infuse your preparations with personal touches sentiments that evoke familiarity and warmth. Include items that hold sentimental value, such as a cherished blanket, a photograph, or a handwritten note to your baby.

Involve Your Partner

Preparing your nest is a collaborative endeavor that involves both you and your partner. Engage in the process together, sharing your ideas, preferences, and aspirations for your baby's living space. Packing the hospital bag can be a bonding experience, as you discuss the items that will accompany you on this transformative journey.

The Journey of Preparation Continues

As you navigate the realm of preparing your nest, remember that these practical preparations are a tangible expression of your readiness to welcome your baby. Your living space becomes a canvas for cherished memories, and your hospital bag holds the promise of the moments that lie ahead.

In the chapters that follow, we will delve deeper into the multifaceted landscape of pregnancy, exploring the emotional preparations for childbirth, the art of bonding with your baby, and the transition into motherhood. We will unveil the practices that support a positive birth experience, offer guidance for early parenting, and provide insights into the incredible journey of nurturing and raising a child.

As you continue on this remarkable journey, may your living space be a haven of comfort, may your hospital bag carry the essentials of love, and may your preparations reflect the beauty of anticipation. Your journey is a symphony of readiness, a dance of nesting, and a tapestry of preparation.

With a heart full of anticipation and a spirit full of readiness, let us navigate the terrain of preparing your nest—a terrain that reflects the art of anticipation and the beauty of welcome.

Chapter 8:

Doctor's Appointments and Prenatal Care

Choosing the Right Healthcare Provider. Navigating Prenatal Tests and Screenings.

In the grand tapestry of pregnancy, healthcare appointments emerge as the threads that weave together the journey of nurturing life. Each appointment is a milestone a moment of connection, guidance, and insight that shapes your path toward motherhood. Central to this journey is the act of choosing the right healthcare provider and navigating the landscape of prenatal tests and screenings. Welcome to the realm of doctor's appointments and prenatal care a journey that explores the significance of your healthcare team and guides you through the maze of medical assessments, ensuring that you receive the best care possible.

Choosing the Right Healthcare Provider

Selecting a healthcare provider is a momentous decision a choice that influences your pregnancy journey and the care you receive. Your healthcare provider becomes a trusted companion a guide who offers medical expertise, answers your questions, and supports you throughout your pregnancy and beyond.

Types of Healthcare Providers

The array of healthcare providers available to expectant mothers includes obstetricians, midwives, family practitioners, and nurse practitioners. Each type of provider brings a unique approach to prenatal care, and your choice should align with your preferences, values, and medical needs.

Obstetricians: Specialized Expertise

Obstetricians are medical doctors who specialize in pregnancy and childbirth. They offer a high level of medical expertise and are equipped to handle both routine pregnancies and high-risk situations. Obstetricians work closely with a team of medical professionals to ensure comprehensive care.

Midwives: Holistic Care

Midwives offer a holistic approach to pregnancy and childbirth, focusing on the emotional, physical, and social aspects of your experience. They often emphasize natural childbirth and provide personalized support during labor. Midwives are particularly well-suited for low-risk pregnancies.

Family Practitioners and Nurse Practitioners: Comprehensive Care

Family practitioners and nurse practitioners offer comprehensive healthcare services, including prenatal care. They are trained to address a wide range of medical needs and can provide integrated care for both you and your baby.

Factors to Consider

When choosing a healthcare provider, consider factors such as their approach to care, their availability, and their compatibility with your preferences. Some questions to consider include:

- What is their philosophy on childbirth and prenatal care?

- Do they offer the type of care you are seeking (e.g., natural, medical, collaborative)?

- What is their communication style, and do you feel comfortable discussing your concerns with them?

- Are they part of a larger healthcare team that can provide comprehensive support?

Navigating Prenatal Tests and Screenings

The landscape of prenatal tests and screenings is a tapestry of medical assessments a mosaic that offers insights into your health and the well-being of your baby. Navigating this terrain involves understanding the purpose of various tests, making informed decisions, and actively participating in your care.

First Trimester: Establishing the Baseline

During the first trimester, your healthcare provider

will conduct a series of tests and screenings to establish a baseline of your health and to assess potential risks. These may include:

- **Blood Tests**: Blood tests measure markers such as your blood type, Rh factor, and immunity to certain infections. They also provide insights into your iron levels and blood sugar.

- **Ultrasound**: An early ultrasound, known as a dating ultrasound, helps determine your due date and provides a first glimpse of your baby's development.

- **Nuchal Translucency Screening:** This test assesses the risk of chromosomal abnormalities, such as Down syndrome.

Second Trimester: Delving Deeper

As your pregnancy progresses, your healthcare provider will continue to monitor your health and your baby's development. Second-trimester tests may include:

- **Maternal Serum Screening**: Also known as the quad screen, this blood test assesses the risk of chromosomal abnormalities and neural tube defects.

- **Anatomy Ultrasound**: This detailed ultrasound evaluates your baby's anatomy and checks for any structural abnormalities.

Third Trimester: Preparing for Birth

In the final trimester, the focus shifts toward preparing for labor and birth. Tests and screenings during this phase may include:

- **Group B Streptococcus (GBS) Screening**: This test determines whether you carry GBS bacteria, which can be passed to the baby during childbirth.

- **Non-Stress Test**: This test monitors your baby's heart rate in response to movement.

- **Biophysical Profile**: This test combines ultrasound and a non-stress test to assess your baby's well-being.

Informed Decision-Making and Participation

Navigating prenatal tests and screenings involves a balance between gathering information and making informed decisions. Your healthcare provider will guide you through the purpose, benefits, and potential risks of each test, allowing you to make choices that align with your preferences and values.

Active Engagement

Participating actively in your prenatal care is an empowering act one that enhances your understanding of your health and your baby's well-being. Ask questions, seek clarification, and express your concerns openly with your healthcare provider. Engaging in discussions about prenatal tests and screenings ensures that you're well-informed and that your care is tailored to your individual needs.

The Journey of Care and Understanding Continues

As you navigate the landscape of doctor's appointments and prenatal care, remember that these moments of connection and assessment are integral to your journey. Your healthcare provider becomes a

trusted partner a guide who supports you in making informed decisions and ensures your health and well-being throughout pregnancy and beyond.

In the chapters that follow, we will delve deeper into the multifaceted landscape of pregnancy, exploring the emotional preparations for childbirth, the art of bonding with your baby, and the transition into motherhood. We will unveil the practices that support a positive birth experience, offer guidance for early parenting, and provide insights into the incredible journey of nurturing and raising a child.

As you continue on this remarkable journey, may your healthcare appointments be moments of connection and understanding, may your decisions be rooted in informed choices, and may your prenatal care reflect the commitment to your well-being. Your journey is a symphony of care, a dance of understanding, and a tapestry of empowerment.

With a heart full of engagement and a spirit full of understanding, let us navigate the terrain of doctor's appointments and prenatal care a terrain that reflects the beauty of informed decisions and the art of care.

Chapter 9:

Bonding with Your Baby: Connecting Before Birth

The Magic of Fetal Development. Communicating and Bonding with Your Baby.

In the breathtaking symphony of pregnancy, a profound connection unfolds a connection that transcends the physical realm and dances in the realm of heart and soul. This connection, forged through the magic of fetal development, is a tapestry of wonder, awe, and anticipation. As you journey toward motherhood, the act of bonding with your baby before birth becomes a poignant expression of love and connection. Welcome to the realm of bonding with your baby a journey that explores the intricate dance of fetal development and guides you in fostering a profound connection with the life growing within you.

The Magic of Fetal Development

Within the cocoon of your womb, an extraordinary journey of creation and growth takes place a journey that unveils the miraculous process of fetal development. From the moment of conception to the exquisite tapestry of organs, senses, and limbs, your baby's growth is a symphony of transformation a dance of life that is as intricate as it is awe-inspiring.

Conception: The Spark of Life

The journey of fetal development begins with the miraculous spark of conception an alchemical union of egg and sperm that carries the blueprint of life. As the fertilized egg divides and multiplies, it forms a blastocyst that implants itself in the lining of your uterus a process that marks the inception of a new life.

The Dance of Cells and Organs

From the moment of implantation, the embryo embarks on a symphonic journey of cell division and differentiation. Each cell carries a unique role and purpose, eventually forming the foundation of your baby's organs, systems, and structures. The heart begins to beat, the brain takes shape, and the skeleton forms a choreography of life orchestrated by the genetic masterpiece within.

Sensory Marvels

As the weeks progress, your baby's senses come alive a symphony of sensory marvels that unfold within the sanctuary of your womb. Your baby's sense of touch develops as early as 8 weeks, followed by the emergence of taste, smell, and hearing. By the second trimester, your baby can hear the rhythm of your heartbeat, the melody of your voice, and the external sounds of the world.

Communicating and Bonding with Your Baby

The journey of bonding with your baby before birth is a sacred dance a dance that nurtures your connection, communicates your love, and fosters a sense of presence between you and your little one. While your baby may not understand language in the traditional sense, the energy, tone, and intention behind your communication are woven into the fabric of your relationship.

The Language of Touch

Touch is a universal language one that transcends words and speaks directly to the heart. Place your hands gently on your belly, and feel the contours of your baby's presence. Your touch offers reassurance and warmth, a tangible expression of love that your baby can feel. As you connect through touch, notice your baby's responses a gentle flutter or a subtle shift that signifies the presence of life.

The Melody of Your Voice

Your voice is a soothing melody a lullaby that cradles your baby's spirit. Engage in conversations with your baby, sharing your thoughts, hopes, and dreams. Read aloud, sing, or simply speak from your heart. Your voice carries the vibration of your emotions and intentions, creating a harmonious connection between you and your baby.

The Dance of Movement

As you move and engage in daily activities, your baby experiences a dance of movement a sensation of being held and swayed within the safety of your womb. Pay attention to your baby's reactions to movement notice if your baby responds with gentle kicks or changes in position. Your movements become a choreography of connection, a dance that mirrors the rhythms of your bond.

Creating Rituals of Connection

Fostering a deep bond with your baby is an intentional practice one that involves creating rituals of connection. These rituals become a bridge between your world and the world of your baby, an avenue for communication and love.

Quiet Moments of Presence

Set aside quiet moments each day to connect with your baby. Find a comfortable space where you can sit or lie down, and close your eyes. Take a few deep breaths to center yourself, and place your hands on your belly. In the stillness, allow yourself to connect with the energy of your baby, tuning into the sensations and emotions that arise.

Guided Meditation and Visualization

Guided meditation and visualization can be powerful tools for deepening your bond with your baby. Envision a serene and safe space where you and your baby are connected in love and light. Imagine your baby's presence, and visualize a gentle exchange of energy between you. This practice not only nurtures your bond but also offers moments of tranquility and relaxation.

The Dance of Connection Continues

As you journey through the landscape of bonding with your baby before birth, remember that this connection is a sacred dance a dance that transcends time and space, a dance that nourishes both your heart and the spirit of your little one.

In the chapters that follow, we will delve deeper into the multifaceted landscape of pregnancy, exploring the emotional preparations for childbirth, the transition into motherhood, and the art of nurturing your well-being. We will unveil the practices that support a positive birth experience, offer guidance for early parenting, and provide insights into the incredible journey of nurturing and raising a child.

As you continue on this remarkable journey, may your bond with your baby be a source of strength, may your communication be a melody

of love, and may your connection be a tapestry of wonder. Your journey is a symphony of presence, a dance of connection, and a tapestry of love.

With a heart full of connection and a spirit full of wonder, let us navigate the terrain of bonding with your baby a terrain that reflects the beauty of presence and the art of love.

Chapter 10:

Coping with Pregnancy Discomforts

Morning Sickness and Other Common Ailments. Remedies for Aches, Pains, and Sleeplessness.

In the exquisite tapestry of pregnancy, the journey is often accompanied by a symphony of sensations some enchanting, others challenging. As your body undergoes profound transformations to nurture the life growing within you, you may encounter an array of discomforts that are as varied as they are temporary. Coping with these discomforts becomes an act of self-care and resilience, a practice that nurtures your well-being and supports your journey toward motherhood. Welcome to the realm of coping with pregnancy discomforts a journey that explores the common ailments, offers remedies for aches and pains, and guides you in finding comfort and relief amidst the shifts and changes.

Morning Sickness and Other Common Ailments

The early days of pregnancy often unfold in a haze of wonder and tenderness a period marked by the emergence of morning sickness and other common ailments. While these discomforts may challenge your well-being, they are also a testament to the incredible journey of nurturing life.

Morning Sickness: Navigating Nausea

Morning sickness, often experienced in the early stages of pregnancy, is a rite of passage that showcases the incredible hormonal shifts occurring within your body. Nausea and vomiting can vary in intensity, and the triggers may differ from woman to woman. While morning sickness is temporary, its impact can be eased through mindful strategies:

- **Small, Frequent Meals**: Consuming small, nutrient-rich meals throughout the day can help stabilize blood sugar levels and reduce the likelihood of nausea.

- **Ginger and Lemon**: Ginger and lemon are known for their anti-nausea properties. Sip ginger tea, add fresh ginger to your meals, or enjoy a slice of lemon in warm water.

- **Hydration**: Staying hydrated is essential. Sip water, herbal teas, and clear broths to maintain hydration.

- **Avoid Triggers**: Identify and avoid triggers that exacerbate nausea. Strong odors, certain foods, and stuffy environments may contribute to feelings of sickness.

Fatigue: Resting and Nurturing

Fatigue is a common companion during pregnancy a gentle reminder that your body is working tirelessly to nurture your baby. Embrace rest and prioritize self-care to navigate fatigue:

- **Naps**: Allow yourself to rest when needed. Short naps during the day can provide a boost of energy.

- **Prioritize Sleep**: Ensure a comfortable sleep environment by using pillows to support your body. Establish a bedtime routine that promotes relaxation.

Nasal Congestion and Bleeding Gums

Hormonal changes during pregnancy can lead to nasal congestion and bleeding gums. Use saline nasal sprays to ease congestion, and maintain good oral hygiene to manage bleeding gums.

Heartburn and Indigestion

As your uterus expands, it can push against your stomach and lead to heartburn and indigestion. Eat smaller meals, avoid spicy and acidic foods, and consider elevating your upper body while sleeping to alleviate symptoms.

Remedies for Aches, Pains, and Sleeplessness

The shifts in your body's structure and the growing weight of your baby can lead to aches, pains, and sleeplessness. Navigating these discomforts requires a holistic approach one that combines physical remedies with self-care practices.

Back Pain: Gentle Movement and Support

Back pain is a common complaint during pregnancy, particularly in the lower back. Engage in gentle exercises such as prenatal yoga, which strengthens the muscles that support your back. Use supportive pillows while sleeping, and practice good posture during daily activities.

Sciatica: Easing Nerve Pain

Sciatica, characterized by pain radiating along the sciatic nerve, can occur due to pressure on the nerve from the growing uterus. Gentle stretches, warm compresses, and prenatal massages can provide relief. Consult your healthcare provider before trying any new remedies.

Swelling and Edema

Swelling in the ankles, feet, and hands is a result of fluid retention. Elevate your feet whenever possible, wear comfortable shoes, and avoid standing for prolonged periods.

Sleeplessness: Cultivating Relaxation

Sleeplessness can be attributed to a combination of physical discomfort and the anticipation of motherhood. Establish a soothing bedtime routine, engage in relaxation techniques such as deep breathing or meditation, and create a comfortable sleep environment.

The Landscape of Self-Care

Coping with pregnancy discomforts is a journey of self-care a journey that requires tenderness, patience, and a deep connection with your body. As you navigate these discomforts, remember that your well-being is a priority, and nurturing yourself supports the health of both you and your baby.

Listening to Your Body

Your body is a remarkable compass one that communicates its needs and responses. Tune into your body's signals, and honor its messages. If discomfort persists or becomes overwhelming, consult your healthcare provider for guidance and support.

The Journey of Self-Care Continues

As you journey through the landscape of coping with pregnancy discomforts, remember that self-care is an art a practice that reflects your resilience and compassion for yourself and your baby.

In the chapters that follow, we will delve deeper into the multifaceted landscape of pregnancy, exploring the emotional preparations for childbirth, the transition into motherhood, and the art of nurturing your well-being. We will unveil the practices that support a positive birth experience, offer guidance for early parenting, and provide insights into the incredible journey of nurturing and raising a child.

As you continue on this remarkable journey, may your self-care practices be a sanctuary of comfort, may your remedies be a source of relief, and may your well-being be a tapestry of resilience. Your journey is a symphony of self-love, a dance of compassion, and a tapestry of care.

With a heart full of tenderness and a spirit full of resilience, let us navigate the terrain of coping with pregnancy discomforts—a terrain that reflects the beauty of self-care and the art of nurturing.

Chapter 11:

Understanding Labor and Childbirth

The Stages of Labor: What to Expect. Creating a Birth Plan.

In the breathtaking journey of pregnancy, the crescendo of anticipation and wonder leads to a transformative moment the arrival of your baby. Labor and childbirth are the culminating chapters of this remarkable narrative, a symphony of strength, resilience, and the miracle of life. Understanding the stages of labor, preparing for the unpredictable, and creating a birth plan become essential components of your journey toward motherhood. Welcome to the realm of understanding labor and childbirth a journey that explores the progression of labor, guides you through the creation of a birth plan, and empowers you to navigate this sacred threshold with confidence and grace.

The Stages of Labor: What to Expect

Labor is a testament to the incredible strength

and endurance of the human body a symphony of contractions, movements, and emotions that mark the journey toward childbirth. Understanding the stages of labor empowers you to navigate this transformative process with knowledge and readiness.

Stage 1: Early Labor

Early labor is a gentle prelude to the more intense stages that follow. Contractions become regular but are generally manageable. This stage may last for several hours or even days, during which your cervix begins to dilate and efface.

Stage 2: Active Labor

Active labor is characterized by more intense and frequent contractions. Your cervix continues to dilate, and your baby's head descends further into the birth canal. The intensity of contractions requires your full attention, and this is typically when you head to the hospital or birthing center.

Stage 3: Transition

Transition is the most challenging and intense phase of labor. Contractions peak in intensity and frequency, and your cervix completes its dilation. Emotions may be heightened, and you might experience self-doubt and exhaustion. Transition is often brief but leads to the final stage of labor.

Stage 4: Second Stage of Labor

The second stage of labor is the moment of birth the culmination of your journey. Your body works in harmony to guide your baby through the birth canal. With each contraction, your baby advances until the head crowns. After the head emerges, the rest of your baby's body follows, completing the incredible journey of childbirth.

Stage 5: Third Stage of Labor

The third stage involves the delivery of the placenta a moment of completion and transition. Your healthcare provider will guide you through this phase, ensuring that all remnants of the placenta are safely removed.

Creating a Birth Plan

Crafting a birth plan is an act of preparation and intention a document that outlines your preferences, desires, and choices for your birthing experience. While childbirth is inherently unpredictable, a birth plan offers a guiding light that empowers you to make informed decisions.

Exploring Your Options

Before creating a birth plan, take time to explore the options available to you. Consider factors such as the location of birth (hospital, birthing center, home), pain management preferences, and the presence of a support person during labor.

Component of a Birth Plan

A birth plan typically includes:

- **Labor Preferences**: Outline your preferences for pain management, movement during labor, and the use of interventions such as induction or augmentation.

- **Support Team**: Specify who you would like to be present during labor and childbirth a partner, family member, or doula.

- **Environment:** Express your desires for the birthing environment, including preferences for lighting, music, and comfort measures.

- **Medical Interventions**: Detail your preferences regarding interventions such as fetal monitoring, episiotomy, and Cesarean birth. Remember that flexibility is key, as unexpected situations may arise.

- **Postpartum Care**: Consider your preferences for immediate postpartum care, including skin-to-skin contact, delayed cord clamping, and breastfeeding.

- **Emergency Scenarios**: Acknowledge that unforeseen circumstances might arise. Outline your preferences in emergency situations, such as a Cesarean birth.

Empowering Your Birth Experience

While a birth plan provides a framework for your desires, it's important to remain flexible and open to the unpredictability of childbirth. Empower yourself by:

- **Educating Yourself**: Learn about the labor process, pain management options, and potential interventions. Knowledge is your ally.

- **Communicating with Your Healthcare Provider**: Share your birth plan with your healthcare provider, and discuss your preferences. Their expertise can guide your decisions and provide valuable insights.

- **Cultivating Mindfulness**: Practice mindfulness techniques to stay present and centered during labor.

Breathing exercises, visualization, and relaxation techniques can ease tension and anxiety.

The Journey of Empowerment Continues

As you navigate the landscape of understanding labor and childbirth, remember that this journey is a symphony of strength, a dance of readiness, and a tapestry of transformation.

In the chapters that follow, we will delve deeper into the multifaceted landscape of pregnancy, exploring the emotional preparations for childbirth, the transition into motherhood, and the art of nurturing your well-being. We will unveil the practices that support a positive birth experience, offer guidance for early parenting, and provide insights into the incredible journey of nurturing and raising a child.

As you continue on this remarkable journey, may your understanding of labor be a source of empowerment, may your birth plan reflect your desires, and may your journey through childbirth be one of strength and grace. Your journey is a symphony of readiness, a dance of choices, and a tapestry of transformation.

With a heart full of empowerment and a spirit full of grace, let us navigate the terrain of understanding labor and childbirth a terrain that reflects the beauty of preparation and the art of empowerment.

Chapter 12:

Preparing for Delivery Day

Packing for the Hospital: Essentials and Comforts. Emotional Readiness for Labor.

As the final crescendo of pregnancy draws near, the anticipation of delivery day becomes a tapestry woven with excitement, preparation, and a touch of trepidation. The day you meet your baby is a milestone of profound significance a culmination of months of nurturing, growth, and transformation. Preparing for delivery day involves a dance of practicality and emotion a choreography that encompasses packing for the hospital and nurturing your emotional readiness for labor. Welcome to the realm of preparing for delivery day a journey that guides you through essentials for your hospital bag, supports your emotional well-being, and empowers you to greet the transformative moment with courage and grace.

Packing for the Hospital: Essentials and Comforts

As you embark on the journey to the birthing center

or hospital, your bag becomes a treasure trove of essentials and comforts a collection of items that will support you during labor and postpartum recovery. Thoughtful packing ensures that you have what you need to navigate this profound experience with comfort and ease.

Essential Items

- **Birth Plan and Medical Documents**: Ensure you have a printed copy of your birth plan, insurance information, and any necessary medical documents.

- **Identification and Hospital Registration**: Keep your photo ID and hospital registration information easily accessible.

- **Comfortable Clothing**: Pack loose, comfortable clothing for labor, such as a loose-fitting nightgown or robe. Consider packing a change of clothes for after delivery.

- **Slippers and Socks**: Comfortable slippers or socks can

provide warmth and comfort during your stay.

- **Toiletries**: Bring travel-sized toiletries, including a toothbrush, toothpaste, shampoo, and lip balm. Hair ties or headbands can also be helpful.

- **Personal Items**: Pack your glasses or contacts, if you wear them, along with any personal items that bring you comfort.

- **Snacks and Drinks**: Consider packing snacks and drinks that provide sustenance during labor. Clear liquids and easily digestible snacks are ideal.

Comfort Items

- **Pillow and Blanket**: Bringing your own pillow and blanket can provide a sense of comfort and familiarity.

- **Entertainment**: Pack a book, magazine, or other form of entertainment to help pass the time during early labor.

- **Electronic Devices**: Don't forget your phone, charger, and headphones. Music or calming apps can help create a soothing atmosphere.

- **Camera or Camcorder**: If you wish to capture the special moments, ensure you have a camera or camcorder and a fully charged battery.

Emotional Readiness for Labor

While the practical aspects of packing for the hospital are important, emotional readiness for labor holds equal significance. Labor is a journey that unfolds on multiple levels physical, emotional, and spiritual. Preparing emotionally allows you to navigate the intensity of labor with grace and presence.

Cultivating Emotional Resilience

- **Mindful Breathing:** Practice mindful breathing

exercises to stay centered and calm. Breathing deeply during contractions can ease tension and anxiety.

- **Visualizations**: Engage in visualizations that align with your birth experience. Envision a calm, serene space where you feel supported and safe.

- **Affirmations**: Create affirmations that resonate with you and affirm your strength. Repeat these affirmations to yourself during labor as a source of empowerment.

Nurturing Support and Connection

- **Partner Support:** If you have a partner or support person, discuss their role and preferences during labor. Their presence can be a source of comfort and reassurance.

- **Communicate Your Needs**: Express your needs and preferences to your healthcare team. Open communication ensures that your desires are respected.

- **Embrace Vulnerability**: Labor is a journey of surrender and vulnerability. Embrace the waves of sensation as a powerful testament to your strength.

The Landscape of Emotional Preparation

Emotional readiness for labor is a journey that embraces the spectrum of human emotions the highs, the lows, and the moments of quiet strength. As you prepare for delivery day, remember that your emotional well-being is a priority.

Journaling and Reflection

Consider keeping a journal in the days leading up to delivery. Write about your hopes, fears, and expectations. Reflect on your journey toward motherhood and your feelings as you approach this transformative moment.

Self-Compassion and Acceptance

Nurturing emotional readiness involves embracing self-compassion and acceptance. Understand that each labor experience is unique, and there is no "right" or "wrong" way to feel. Allow yourself to experience a range of emotions without judgment.

The Journey of Emotional Readiness Continues

As you navigate the landscape of preparing for delivery day, remember that emotional preparation is a dance of presence, a symphony of courage, and a tapestry of readiness.

In the chapters that follow, we will delve deeper into the multifaceted landscape of pregnancy, exploring the emotional preparations for childbirth, the transition into motherhood, and the art of nurturing your well-being. We will unveil the practices that support a positive birth experience, offer guidance for early parenting, and provide insights into the incredible journey of nurturing and raising a child.

As you continue on this remarkable journey, may your emotional readiness be a source of strength, may your bag be a reflection of comfort, and may your heart be open to the transformative magic of delivery day. Your journey is a symphony of presence, a dance of emotion, and a tapestry of courage.

With a heart full of readiness and a spirit full of grace, let us navigate the terrain of preparing for delivery day a terrain that reflects the beauty of emotional presence and the art of preparation.

Chapter 13:

Cesarean Birth: What You Need to Know

When C-Section Becomes Necessary. Recovery and Navigating Post-Cesarean Care.

In the intricate tapestry of childbirth, the journey can take unexpected turns-turns that may lead to a Cesarean birth, also known as a C-section. While the anticipation of a vaginal birth often takes center stage, understanding the nuances of a Cesarean birth is an essential aspect of childbirth education. When circumstances necessitate a C-section, navigating the process with knowledge and readiness empowers you to embrace this alternative path with courage and grace. Welcome to the realm of Cesarean birth a journey that explores when a C-section becomes necessary, guides you through recovery, and offers insights into post-Cesarean care as you embark on the next chapter of motherhood.

When C-Section Becomes Necessary

A Cesarean birth is a surgical procedure in which

your baby is delivered through an incision made in your abdomen and uterus. While the majority of births occur vaginally, there are instances where a C-section becomes the safest option for you and your baby. Understanding the scenarios that may lead to a C-section prepares you for potential outcomes and decisions that may arise.

Medical Indications for a C-Section

- **Breech Presentation**: If your baby is positioned feet or buttocks first (breech), a C-section may be recommended to ensure a safe delivery.

- **Placenta Previa**: When the placenta partially or completely covers the cervix, a C-section may be necessary to prevent bleeding complications.

- **Fetal Distress**: If your baby's heart rate shows signs of distress during labor, a C-section may be performed to ensure your baby's well-being.

- **Labor Complications**: Prolonged labor, failure to

progress, or concerns about the baby's ability to tolerate labor may lead to a C-section.

- **Multiple Gestation**: If you are carrying multiples (twins, triplets), a C-section may be recommended based on factors such as positioning and number of babies.

- **Maternal Health Conditions**: Certain maternal health conditions, such as high blood pressure or active genital herpes, may necessitate a C-section.

Recovery and Navigating Post-Cesarean Care

Recovery after a Cesarean birth involves both physical healing and emotional adjustment. Navigating post-Cesarean care with self-compassion and awareness supports your well-being and sets the stage for your transition into motherhood.

Physical Recovery

- **Hospital Stay**: After a C-section, you will likely spend a few days in the hospital for monitoring and recovery. Pain medication and support garments may be provided.

- **Incision Care**: Proper care of the incision site is essential for preventing infection and promoting healing. Keep the incision clean and dry, and follow your healthcare provider's instructions.

- **Physical Activity**: Initially, your activity will be limited. Gradually incorporate gentle movements and walking into your routine as advised by your healthcare provider.

- **Pain Management**: Pain and discomfort are normal after a C-section. Your healthcare provider will provide guidance on pain management options, which may include medication and non-pharmacological techniques.

Emotional Recovery

- **Processing the Experience**: A C-section can bring a range of emotions. Allow yourself to process your feelings and seek support from your partner, family, or a mental health professional if needed.

- **Bonding with Your Baby**: Embrace skin-to-skin contact and breastfeeding as ways to bond with your baby, even after a C-section.

- **Accepting Assistance**: Accepting help from others during your recovery is not a sign of weakness, but an act of self-care. Allow loved ones to support you as you navigate the early days of motherhood.

- **Managing Expectations**: Give yourself permission to adjust your expectations. Recovery after a C-section may require more time and patience than you initially anticipated.

The Landscape of Cesarean Birth and Beyond

A Cesarean birth is a unique path one that intersects with the journey of childbirth and marks the beginning of your role as a mother. As you navigate the landscape of Cesarean birth, remember that your experience is valid, your emotions are valid, and your journey is uniquely yours.

Embracing Your Story

Every birth story is a testament to strength, resilience, and the capacity of the human spirit. Whether your journey unfolds through a vaginal birth or a Cesarean birth, it is a chapter of your life's narrative a chapter that shapes your identity as a mother.

Nurturing Emotional Resilience

Nurturing emotional resilience after a Cesarean birth involves allowing yourself to grieve any unmet expectations while celebrating the safe arrival of your baby. Reach out to support groups, online communities, or healthcare professionals who can provide guidance and connection during your healing process.

The Journey of Cesarean Birth Continues

As you navigate the landscape of Cesarean birth,

remember that your journey is one of

courage, strength, and grace a journey that encompasses both the unexpected and the transformative.

In the chapters that follow, we will delve deeper into the multifaceted landscape of pregnancy, exploring the emotional preparations for childbirth, the transition into motherhood, and the art of nurturing your well-being. We will unveil the practices that support a positive birth experience, offer guidance for early parenting, and provide insights into the incredible journey of nurturing and raising a child.

As you continue on this remarkable journey, may your knowledge be a source of empowerment, may your recovery be a testament to your resilience, and may your heart be open to the beauty of motherhood. Your journey is a symphony of adaptation, a dance of strength, and a tapestry of love.

With a heart full of understanding and a spirit full of

grace, let us navigate the terrain of Cesarean birth a terrain that reflects the beauty of adaptation and the art of embracing change.

Chapter 14:

The Fourth Trimester: Your Body After Birth

Physical and Emotional Changes Postpartum. Healing and Self-Care in the Early Weeks.

In the tender embrace of motherhood, the journey of pregnancy finds its culmination and birth becomes the threshold to a new chapter a chapter often referred to as the fourth trimester. This uncharted territory is a landscape of transformation, a tapestry woven with physical changes, emotional shifts, and the rhythm of healing. As you welcome your baby into the world, you also step into the sacred realm of postpartum the space where your body and soul undergo a journey of restoration, adjustment, and growth. The fourth trimester is a testament to your strength, your adaptability, and your capacity to nurture both your baby and yourself. Welcome to the realm of the fourth trimester a journey that explores the physical and emotional changes postpartum, guides you through healing and self-care in the early weeks, and invites you to embrace the exquisite dance of becoming a mother.

Physical and Emotional Changes Postpartum

The birth of your baby initiates a series of profound shiftsphysically, emotionally, and spiritually. The first weeks after birth are a time of transition a space where you navigate the terrain of change with gentleness, patience, and self-compassion.

Physical Changes

- **Uterine Contractions**: Your uterus contracts as it returns to its pre-pregnancy size. These contractions, known as afterpains, may be accompanied by mild discomfort.

- **Vaginal Bleeding**: Lochia, the postpartum discharge, is a combination of blood, tissue, and mucus. The flow gradually decreases over the course of a few weeks.

- **Breast Changes**: Your breasts undergo changes as they transition from pregnancy to breastfeeding. They may become swollen, tender, and engorged as your milk comes in.

- **Perineal Discomfort**: If you had a vaginal birth, you

may experience perineal discomfort or soreness. Warm compresses, sitz baths, and pain relief measures can provide relief.

Emotional Changes

- **Baby Blues**: It's common to experience mood swings and emotional vulnerability during the early postpartum period. These feelings, often referred to as baby blues, typically resolve on their own.

- **Postpartum Depression and Anxiety**: Some women experience more intense emotional challenges, such as postpartum depression or anxiety. If you find that your emotions are overwhelming or persistent, seek support from your healthcare provider.

- **Adjustment to Motherhood**: Becoming a mother is a profound transformation. Allow yourself time to adjust to your new role and embrace the changes it brings.

Healing and Self-Care in the Early Weeks

As your body and soul embark on the journey of healing, nurturing yourself becomes an act of love for yourself and for your baby. The early weeks of the fourth trimester are a period of cocooning, a time to prioritize rest, recovery, and connection.

Prioritizing Rest

- **Rest When You Can**: Sleep deprivation is a hallmark of early parenthood. Prioritize sleep by resting when your baby sleeps and allowing your partner or loved ones to help with nighttime feedings.

- **Napping**: Short, frequent naps can help alleviate sleep deprivation and restore your energy.

Nourishing Your Body

- **Balanced Nutrition**: Focus on nourishing, nutrient-dense meals that support your healing and provide energy for breastfeeding.

- **Hydration**: Stay hydrated by drinking plenty of water throughout the day.

- **Snacks**: Have nutritious snacks readily available to fuel your body between meals.

Embracing Self-Care

- **Gentle Movement**: Incorporate gentle movement, such as stretching or short walks, to promote circulation and ease stiffness.

- **Pelvic Floor Exercises**: Pelvic floor exercises, also known as Kegels, can aid in pelvic floor recovery.

- **Mindfulness and Relaxation**: Engage in mindfulness practices, deep breathing, or meditation to support emotional well-being.

- **Support System**: Accept help from loved ones and create a support system that allows you to focus on healing and bonding with your baby.

The Landscape of Healing and Growth

The fourth trimester is a sacred space a cocoon where you undergo a journey of healing, restoration, and growth. As you embrace the dance of physical recovery and emotional adjustment, remember that you are not alone on this path.

Creating Sacred Moments

Amidst the busyness of early motherhood, create sacred moments that nourish your soul. Whether it's a quiet cup of tea, a few moments of deep breathing, or a warm bath, these small acts of self-care are a testament to your commitment to your well-being.

Navigating Emotional Terrain

Navigating the emotional terrain of the fourth trimester involves acknowledging the full spectrum of your feelings. Celebrate moments of joy, seek support during moments of vulnerability, and allow yourself to rest in the gentle embrace of self-compassion.

The Journey of Healing Continues

As you navigate the landscape of the fourth trimester, remember that healing is a symphony of tenderness, a dance of self-love, and a tapestry of growth.

In the chapters that follow, we will delve deeper into the multifaceted landscape of motherhood, exploring the art of nurturing your well-being, fostering a deep bond with your baby, and embracing the journey of parenting. We will unveil the practices that support you as a mother, offer guidance for early parenting challenges, and provide insights into the remarkable journey of raising a child.

As you continue on this remarkable journey, may your healing be a source of empowerment, may your self-care be a testament to your strength, and may your heart be open to the exquisite beauty of the fourth trimester. Your journey is a symphony of restoration, a dance of transformation, and a tapestry of love.

With a heart full of healing and a spirit full of grace, let us navigate the terrain of the fourth trimester a terrain that reflects the beauty of self-care and the art of embracing change.

Chapter 15:

Breastfeeding and Bottle-Feeding Essentials

Navigating Feeding Choices and Challenges. Breastfeeding Techniques and Tips.

In the delicate tapestry of early motherhood, the nourishment you provide your baby becomes a thread that weaves through the journey a thread of connection, sustenance, and love. The choice between breastfeeding and bottle-feeding is an intimate decision that embraces your unique circumstances, desires, and the well-being of both you and your baby. As you embark on this chapter of nurturing, it's essential to approach feeding with compassion, preparation, and the knowledge that every path is valid. Welcome to the realm of feeding essentials a journey that navigates feeding choices and challenges, offers insights into breastfeeding techniques and tips, and empowers you to create a nourishing connection that resonates with your heart.

Navigating Feeding Choices and Challenges

The decision to breastfeed or bottle-feed is a deeply personal one, shaped by your individual circumstances, beliefs, and desires. Both paths offer unique benefits and considerations, and your choice is a testament to your dedication to your baby's well-being.

Breastfeeding

- **Benefits**: Breast milk is a miraculous elixir, providing your baby with essential nutrients, immune-boosting properties, and a unique bond. The act of breastfeeding fosters skin-to-skin contact and emotional connection.

- **Challenges**: Breastfeeding may come with challenges such as latch issues, nipple soreness, and supply concerns. Seek support from lactation consultants, healthcare providers, and support groups if you encounter difficulties.

Bottle-Feeding

- **Benefits**: Bottle-feeding provides flexibility, allowing other caregivers to participate in feeding and offering a clear measure of milk intake. It can be a valuable option for those who choose not to breastfeed or encounter challenges with breastfeeding.

- **Challenges**: Preparing formula, sterilizing bottles, and managing feeding routines may involve more planning. Ensuring proper formula selection and bottle hygiene is crucial.

Breastfeeding Techniques and Tips

If you choose to breastfeed, cultivating a positive and comfortable breastfeeding experience is paramount. Understanding techniques, addressing challenges, and seeking support can enhance your breastfeeding journey.

Preparing for Breastfeeding

- **Educate Yourself:** Learn about breastfeeding techniques, proper latch, and positioning. Attend breastfeeding classes and seek advice from lactation consultants.

- **Create a Nurturing Environment**: Designate a comfortable space for breastfeeding. Surround yourself with pillows, water, snacks, and anything else that brings comfort.

Latching and Positioning

- **Proper Latch:** A proper latch is essential for effective breastfeeding. Ensure your baby's mouth covers both your nipple and areola.

- **Positioning**: Experiment with different breastfeeding positions to find the one that works best for you and your baby. Common positions include cradle hold, football hold, and side-lying.

Overcoming Challenges

- **Nipple Soreness**: Use lanolin cream and ensure a proper latch to minimize nipple soreness.

- **Engorgement**: Gentle massage, warm compresses,

and frequent nursing can relieve engorgement.

- **Low Milk Supply**: Stay hydrated, nurse frequently, and consider techniques to boost milk production, such as pumping after feeds.

Nurturing Emotional Connection

Breastfeeding is more than nourishment; it's a symphony of connection and love. Embrace the quiet moments of closeness, gaze into your baby's eyes, and savor the intimacy of this precious bond.

The Dance of Nourishment and Connection

Whether you choose breastfeeding, bottle-feeding, or a combination of both, remember that the essence of feeding is nurturing an act that reflects your love, dedication, and commitment to your baby's well-being.

Flexibility and Adaptability

As you navigate the landscape of feeding, remain

flexible and adaptable. Every feeding journey is unique, and the path may evolve as your baby grows.

Nurturing Connection

Nourishment is an opportunity for connection a dance that transcends feeding itself. Cherish the tender moments, the skin-to-skin contact, and the opportunity to meet your baby's needs with tenderness and love.

The Journey of Nurturing Continues

As you navigate the realm of feeding essentials, remember that the choices you make are a testament to your devotion to your baby's well-being, and that every path is valid.

In the chapters that follow, we will delve deeper into the multifaceted landscape of motherhood, exploring the art of fostering a deep bond with your baby, nurturing your well-being, and embracing the journey of parenting. We will unveil the practices that support you as a mother, offer guidance for early parenting challenges, and provide insights into the remarkable journey of raising a child.

As you continue on this remarkable journey, may your feeding experiences be a source of connection, may your nurturing be a testament to your love, and may your heart be open to the exquisite dance of motherhood. Your journey is a symphony of nourishment, a dance of love, and a tapestry of connection.

With a heart full of dedication and a spirit full of grace, let us navigate the terrain of feeding essentials a terrain that reflects the beauty of choice and the art of nurturing.

Chapter 16:

Newborn Care: From Diapering to Soothing

Diapering, Bathing, and Basic Care. Creating a Safe Sleep Environment.

In the delicate tapestry of early parenthood, caring for your newborn becomes a symphony of tenderness a melody that involves the delicate art of diapering, bathing, and creating a haven of safety for restful sleep. As you embrace the journey of nurturing your baby's needs, you step into a realm of learning, adapting, and discovering the exquisite dance of care. From the soft touch of a clean diaper to the soothing embrace of a warm bath, every moment becomes an opportunity to connect, protect, and guide your baby through the landscape of infancy. Welcome to the realm of newborn care a journey that encompasses diapering, bathing, and basic care, while crafting a haven of safety for peaceful sleep.

Diapering, Bathing, and Basic Care

Caring for your newborn involves a series of daily

rituals that strengthen the bond between you and your baby. From the first diaper change to the gentle bath, each task is an act of love that fosters connection, hygiene, and well-being.

Diapering

- **Gather Supplies**: Before you begin, ensure you have all the necessary supplies within reach clean diapers, wipes, diaper cream, and a change of clothes.

- **Changing Station**: Create a dedicated changing station with a soft changing pad or surface. Keep it stocked with all the essentials.

- **Diapering Technique**: Gently lift your baby's legs to remove the soiled diaper. Wipe the area with a clean wipe, using gentle strokes. For girls, wipe from front to back to prevent infections.

- **Diaper Cream**: If your baby's skin is prone to irritation, apply a thin layer of diaper cream to protect the skin.

- **Fresh Diaper**: Place a clean diaper under your baby and secure it snugly. Dispose of the soiled diaper properly.

Bathing

- **Frequency**: In the early weeks, you don't need to bathe your baby daily. A few times a week is sufficient to keep them clean.

- **Sponge Bath**: In the beginning, you can give your baby a sponge bath using a soft washcloth, warm water, and mild soap.

- **Tub Bath**: As your baby grows and their umbilical cord stump falls off, you can transition to tub baths. Fill a baby bathtub with a few inches of warm water and gently bathe your baby.

- **Support and Comfort**: Always support your baby's head and neck during the bath. Keep the room warm and free from drafts.

- **Pat Dry**: After the bath, gently pat your baby dry with a soft towel, paying special attention to skin folds.

Creating a Safe Sleep Environment

Creating a safe sleep environment is paramount to your baby's well-being. A safe sleep space reduces the risk of Sudden Infant Death Syndrome (SIDS) and ensures your baby sleeps soundly.

Safe Sleep Practices

- **Back to Sleep**: Always place your baby on their back for sleep, both for naps and nighttime sleep.

- **Firm Mattress**: Use a firm and flat mattress designed for infants. Avoid soft bedding, pillows, and stuffed animals in the crib.

- **Crib Safety**: Keep the crib free from clutter and ensure that there are no gaps between the mattress and the crib frame.

- **Temperature Control**: Keep the room at a comfortable temperature, and dress your baby in light sleep clothing.

- **No Smoking:** Keep your baby's sleep environment smoke-free.

The Dance of Connection and Safety

As you navigate the realm of newborn care, remember that each task from diapering to bathing is an opportunity to connect with your baby and ensure their well-being.

Listening to Your Baby

Pay attention to your baby's cues and preferences. Some babies enjoy bath time as a soothing experience, while others prefer it quick and efficient. Similarly, some babies love being diaper-free during playtime.

Soothing Touch

Infant care involves a symphony of touch a gentle massage during diaper changes, the caress of a soft towel after a bath, and the soothing embrace of swaddling for sleep.

The Journey of Care and Connection Continues

As you navigate the landscape of newborn care, remember that every touch, every diaper change, and every bath is an act of love a melody that reflects your devotion to your baby's well-being.

In the chapters that follow, we will delve deeper into the multifaceted landscape of early parenting, exploring the art of nurturing your well-being, fostering a deep bond with your baby, and embracing the journey of raising a child. We will unveil the practices that support you as a parent, offer guidance for early parenting challenges, and provide insights into the remarkable journey of parenting.

As you continue on this remarkable journey, may

your caregiving be a source of connection, may your nurturing be a testament to your love, and may your heart be open to the exquisite dance of parenthood. Your journey is a symphony of care, a dance of connection, and a tapestry of love.

With a heart full of tenderness and a spirit full of grace, let us navigate the terrain of newborn care a terrain that reflects the beauty of nurturing and the art of parenting.

Chapter 17:

Embracing Parenthood: Navigating the New Roles

From Partners to Parents: Strengthening Bonds. Balancing Work, Parenthood, and Self-Care.

In the heartwarming tapestry of parenthood, the journey takes a transformative turn partners become parents, and the landscape shifts to accommodate new roles, responsibilities, and a profound bond that deepens with each passing day. Navigating the transition from partners to parents is a remarkable dance a symphony of love, growth, and adaptation that requires intention, communication, and a commitment to nurturing both your child and your partnership. As you embrace the journey of parenthood, the art of balancing work, family, and self-care takes center stage, inviting you to harmonize the different facets of your life. Welcome to the realm of embracing parenthood a journey that explores strengthening bonds as partners turned parents, and offers insights into balancing the intricate tapestry of work, parenthood, and self-care.

From Partners to Parents: Strengthening Bonds

The transition from being partners to becoming parents is a beautiful metamorphosis that invites you to deepen your connection, communication, and shared journey. As you navigate this transition, remember that your partnership is the foundation upon which your family is built.

Embracing Change

- **Communication:** Open and honest communication is essential during this transition. Share your feelings, concerns, and aspirations with each other.

- **Prioritizing Your Relationship:** While parenthood requires attention, it's crucial to continue nurturing your relationship. Plan date nights, engage in shared hobbies, and celebrate each other's achievements.

Division of Labor

- **Shared Responsibilities:** Discuss and agree upon how you will divide parenting responsibilities, household chores, and work commitments. Flexibility is key as you adapt to your baby's needs.

- **Supporting Each Other**: Acknowledge that parenting can be demanding. Support each other emotionally and practically to ensure both partners feel valued and cared for.

Balancing Work, Parenthood, and Self-Care

As parents, you navigate a delicate dance of balancing work commitments, nurturing your child's well-being, and maintaining your own self-care. Finding harmony among these demands requires mindful planning, setting boundaries, and a commitment to your own well-being.

Managing Work Commitments

- **Open Communication**: Communicate with your employer about your parental leave, flexible work options, and any adjustments you may need.

- **Prioritizing Tasks**: Focus on prioritizing tasks and setting realistic goals. Be open about your availability and make use of tools that enhance productivity.

Nurturing Your Child's Well-Being

- **Quality Time**: Create quality moments with your child by engaging in activities that promote bonding and exploration.

- **Routines**: Establish routines that provide structure and predictability for your child, making transitions smoother.

Self-Care for Parents

- **Boundaries**: Set clear boundaries between work and personal time. Designate specific times for work-related tasks and family activities.

- **Me Time**: Allocate time for self-care activities that recharge your energy and nourish your soul. Whether it's reading, exercise, or creative pursuits, prioritize activities that bring you joy.

- **Support System**: Lean on your support system—

whether it's family, friends, or hired help to share the load and create pockets of time for self-care.

The Dance of Balance and Connection

As you navigate the intricate dance of embracing parenthood, remember that balance is a symphony of intention, communication, and adaptability a dance that transforms partners into co-parents while preserving the essence of your partnership.

Shared Moments

Celebrate the small victories, the shared laughter, and the tender moments as you navigate this transformative journey together.

Honoring Individual Identities

While the role of parenthood is all-encompassing, remember that you are still individuals with your own aspirations, dreams, and interests. Nurture your individual identities to enrich your partnership.

The Journey of Parenthood Continues

As you navigate the realm of embracing parenthood, remember that the journey is a testament to your love, commitment, and dedication to your child, your partnership, and yourselves.

In the chapters that follow, we will delve deeper into the multifaceted landscape of parenting, exploring the art of fostering a deep bond with your child, nurturing your well-being, and embracing the journey of raising a child. We will unveil the practices that support you as parents, offer guidance for parenting challenges, and provide insights into the remarkable journey of raising a child.

As you continue on this remarkable journey, may your partnership thrive, may your self-care flourish, and may your hearts be open to the exquisite dance of parenthood. Your journey is a symphony of connection, a dance of balance, and a tapestry of love.

With a heart full of dedication and a spirit full of grace, let us navigate the terrain of embracing parenthood a terrain that reflects the beauty of partnership and the art of nurturing.

Chapter 18:

Postpartum Fitness and Wellness

Easing Back into Physical Activity. Postpartum Mental Health and Well-being.

In the tender tapestry of early motherhood, the journey of postpartum fitness and wellness unfolds a journey that encompasses not only the physical aspects of recovery but also the profound importance of nurturing your mental and emotional well-being. The art of easing back into physical activity after childbirth and fostering postpartum mental health are intertwined, reflecting the delicate dance of self-care, adaptation, and the celebration of the remarkable journey you've embarked upon. As you embrace the path of postpartum wellness, you weave a tapestry of strength, resilience, and grace a tapestry that honors the changes within you and guides you toward holistic well-being. Welcome to the realm of postpartum fitness and wellness a journey that explores the gradual return to physical activity and offers insights into nurturing your mental health during this transformative phase.

Easing Back into Physical Activity

The path of postpartum fitness is one that requires patience, gentleness, and a deep respect for your body's journey. As you navigate this terrain, remember that your body has undergone a remarkable transformation, and its needs deserve your understanding and care.

Listening to Your Body

- **Start Gradually**: Begin with gentle movements that honor your body's current state. Walking, stretching, and light yoga can be excellent starting points.

- **Pelvic Floor Exercises**: Engage in pelvic floor exercises to support the recovery of your pelvic muscles. Consult with a physical therapist if needed.

- **Core Activation**: Gradually reintroduce core exercises, focusing on reestablishing a strong foundation. Avoid movements that strain the abdominal muscles.

Nurturing Recovery

- **Hydration and Nutrition**: Stay hydrated and nourish your body with nutrient-dense foods that support healing and energy levels.

- **Rest and Sleep**: Prioritize rest and sleep to aid in your body's recovery. Nap when your baby naps to replenish your energy.

- **Supportive Gear**: Wear supportive clothing and proper footwear during physical activity to prevent discomfort and strain.

Postpartum Mental Health and Well-being

Nurturing your mental and emotional well-being is a cornerstone of postpartum wellness. As you navigate the emotional landscape of early motherhood, remember that seeking support and practicing self-compassion are essential steps toward optimal mental health.

Embracing Emotions

- **Normalize Emotions**: Understand that a range of emotions is common during the postpartum period. Feelings of joy, exhaustion, and vulnerability can coexist.

- **Talk About It**: Openly discuss your feelings with your partner, friends, or a mental health professional. Sharing your experiences can alleviate feelings of isolation.

Practicing Self-Care

- **Self-Compassion**: Treat yourself with the same kindness and understanding you would offer a friend. Embrace imperfection and let go of unrealistic expectations.

- **Mindfulness and Relaxation**: Engage in mindfulness practices, deep breathing, or meditation to alleviate stress and promote emotional well-being.

- **Asking for Help**: Don't hesitate to ask for help when needed. Whether it's childcare, household tasks, or emotional support, your support system is there to assist you.

The Dance of Well-being and Self-Care

As you navigate the delicate terrain of postpartum fitness and wellness, remember that the journey is a testament to your strength, your adaptability, and your commitment to nurturing both your body and your spirit.

Celebrating Progress

Celebrate every step forward on your postpartum fitness journey. Whether it's increasing your daily steps, regaining flexibility, or engaging in a new fitness routine, each achievement is a triumph.

Nurturing Mind, Body, and Soul

Your postpartum wellness journey is a holistic one a journey that nurtures not only your body but also your mind and soul. As you care for your baby, remember to care for yourself with the same devotion.

The Journey of Wellness Continues

As you navigate the realm of postpartum fitness and wellness, remember that the path you tread is a reflection of your commitment to nurturing your body, embracing your emotions, and celebrating the intricate tapestry of motherhood.

In the chapters that follow, we will delve deeper into the multifaceted landscape of parenting, exploring the art of fostering a deep bond with your child, nurturing your well-being, and embracing the journey of raising a child. We will unveil the practices that support you as parents, offer guidance for parenting challenges, and provide insights into the remarkable journey of raising a child.

As you continue on this remarkable journey, may your fitness journey be filled with self-love, may your mental health flourish, and may your heart be open to the exquisite dance of motherhood. Your journey is a symphony of strength, a dance of well-being, and a tapestry of love.

With a heart full of resilience and a spirit full of grace, let us navigate the terrain of postpartum fitness and wellness a terrain that reflects the beauty of self-care and the art of embracing change.

Chapter 19:

Navigating Changes in Relationships

Intimacy and Communication After Baby. Nurturing Your Connection as a Couple.

In the intricate tapestry of parenthood, the dynamics of your relationships undergo a transformation as you navigate the uncharted waters of welcoming a new life into your family. The journey of navigating changes in relationships encompasses the delicate art of nurturing intimacy, fostering open communication, and preserving the connection between you and your partner. As you embrace the role of parents, you're called to simultaneously honor your roles as partners to cultivate a bond that not only weathers the challenges but flourishes amidst the changes. The path to sustaining a strong and loving relationship as you embrace parenthood requires intention, understanding, and a commitment to growth. Welcome to the realm of navigating changes in relationships a journey that explores the evolution of intimacy and communication after having a baby and offers insights into nurturing your connection as a couple.

Intimacy and Communication After Baby

The arrival of a baby introduces a myriad of changes to your daily routine, priorities, and emotions. As you adapt to these changes, nurturing intimacy and maintaining open communication become cornerstones of sustaining a strong and fulfilling relationship.

Embracing New Dynamics

- **Understanding Changes**: Recognize that the changes in your relationship are a natural part of the transition into parenthood. Embrace the shifts with compassion and patience.

- **Prioritizing Time**: Set aside quality time for each other. Whether it's a date night at home or a quiet moment to reconnect, prioritize nurturing your partnership.

Open Communication

- **Check-Ins**: Regularly check in with each other about your feelings, needs, and expectations. Create a safe space where you can openly share your thoughts.

- **Listening**: Practice active listening when your partner expresses themselves. Validate their emotions and offer support.

- **Team Approach**: Approach parenting as a team effort. Collaborate on decisions, share responsibilities, and recognize each other's contributions.

Nurturing Your Connection as a Couple

Nurturing your relationship as a couple amidst the demands of parenthood requires intentional actions that reflect your commitment to each other. The connection you share becomes the foundation upon which your family thrives.

Quality Time

- **Date Nights**: Continue enjoying date nights, even if they're at home. Cook a special meal, watch a movie, or engage in activities that allow you to connect.

- **Shared Hobbies**: Pursue shared hobbies that bring you joy. Whether it's hiking, cooking, or dancing, these activities strengthen your bond.

Physical Intimacy

- **Patience and Understanding**: Understand that physical intimacy may change after having a baby. Communicate openly about your desires, concerns, and any physical changes you're experiencing.

- **Reconnection**: As you feel ready, prioritize reconnecting physically. Be patient and explore new ways to experience intimacy that are comfortable for both partners.

The Dance of Connection and Growth

As you navigate the evolving landscape of relationships after having a baby, remember that the journey is an opportunity to grow individually and as a couple to embrace change while preserving the essence of your bond.

Celebrating Milestones

Celebrate not only your baby's milestones but also the milestones of your relationship. Reflect on the journey you've shared and the growth you've experienced together.

Embracing Vulnerability

Vulnerability is the cornerstone of deepening intimacy. Share your feelings, fears, and aspirations with your partner. By opening up, you invite them to do the same.

The Journey of Connection Continues

As you navigate the realm of navigating changes

in relationships, remember that the path you tread is a reflection of your dedication to fostering love, understanding, and growth within your partnership.

In the chapters that follow, we will delve deeper into the multifaceted landscape of parenting, exploring the art of fostering a deep bond with your child, nurturing your well-being, and embracing the journey of raising a child. We will unveil the practices that support you as parents, offer guidance for parenting challenges, and provide insights into the remarkable journey of raising a child.

As you continue on this remarkable journey, may your connection flourish, may your communication thrive, and may your hearts be open to the exquisite dance of parenthood. Your journey is a symphony of understanding, a dance of growth, and a tapestry of love.

With a heart full of devotion and a spirit full of grace, let us navigate the terrain of navigating changes in relationships a terrain that reflects the beauty of partnership and the art of nurturing.

Chapter 20:

Returning to Work: Balancing Career and Motherhood

partnership and the art of nurturing.

Chapter 20:

Returning to Work: Balancing Career and Motherhood

Back to Work: Tips and Strategies. Exploring Childcare Options.

In the intricate tapestry of motherhood, the moment arrives when you embark on a new chapter the return to work. This journey encompasses the delicate art of transitioning from the cocoon of early motherhood to the world of your career, while navigating the terrain of balancing your professional responsibilities with your role as a mother. As you embrace the dual role of career woman and mother, you step onto a path that requires intention, adaptability, and a commitment to finding harmony between the two facets of your life. The journey of returning to work and balancing career and motherhood is one that calls upon your resilience, organizational skills, and the ability to embrace change. Welcome to the realm of returning to work a journey that explores the strategies for transitioning back to the workplace and offers insights into exploring childcare options that align with your family's needs.

Transitioning Back to Work: Tips and Strategies

The transition from maternity leave to returning to work is a multifaceted journey one that blends the demands of your career with the responsibilities of motherhood. Navigating this journey requires careful planning, a supportive network, and the ability to set realistic expectations for yourself.

Preparation and Planning

- **Early Communication**: Engage in open communication with your employer before your return. Discuss your work schedule, remote work options, and any adjustments you may need.

- **Trial Runs**: Consider doing a few trial runs of your morning routine before your actual return. This helps identify potential challenges and allows you to fine-tune your schedule.

- **Childcare Arrangements**: Research and secure childcare arrangements well in advance. Visit potential daycare centers or interview potential caregivers to ensure a comfortable fit.

Prioritizing Self-Care

- **Rest and Sleep:** Prioritize rest and sleep as you transition back to work. Ensure you're well-rested to manage the demands of both your job and motherhood.

- **Meal Planning**: Plan and prepare meals in advance to simplify your mornings and evenings. This reduces stress and ensures you're nourished throughout the day.

Exploring Childcare Options

Choosing the right childcare option for your family is a crucial decision that impacts both your child's well-being and your peace of mind. Exploring different options and finding the one that aligns with your values and needs is paramount.

Daycare Centers

- **Structured Environment:** Daycare centers offer a structured and educational environment for children, with opportunities for social interaction and learning.

- **Professional Caregivers**: Children are looked after by trained caregivers who follow established routines and offer developmental activities.

In-Home Caregivers

- **Personalized Care**: In-home caregivers provide one-on-one attention and care tailored to your child's individual needs.

- **Familiar Environment:** Your child remains in the comfort of their own home, which can provide a sense of security.

Family and Friends

- **Support System**: Enlisting the help of family members or friends can provide a support system that aligns with your child's needs.

- **Flexibility**: Family and friends may offer more flexible care arrangements, allowing you to customize your child's routine.

The Dance of Juggling Roles

As you navigate the terrain of returning to work and balancing career and motherhood, remember that the journey is an opportunity to embrace your roles as both a professional and a mother to find harmony in the dance of juggling responsibilities.

Finding Balance

Striving for balance doesn't mean achieving perfection in every aspect of your life. Rather, it's about acknowledging the ebb and flow of your roles and making conscious choices that align with your priorities.

Nurturing Your Well-Being

Remember that nurturing your well-being is essential to successfully navigate the dual roles of career and motherhood. Prioritize self-care, seek support when needed, and celebrate your accomplishments.

The Journey of Balance Continues

As you navigate the realm of returning to work and balancing career and motherhood, remember that the path you tread is a reflection of your dedication to your career, your family, and yourself.

In the chapters that precede and follow, we have explored the multifaceted landscape of motherhood, delving into the art of nurturing your well-being, fostering connections, and embracing the remarkable journey of raising a child. We have unveiled the practices that support you as parents, offered guidance for parenting challenges, and provided insights into the extraordinary journey of parenthood.

As you continue on this remarkable journey, may your career flourish, may your family thrive, and may your heart be open to the exquisite dance of balancing career and motherhood. Your journey is a symphony of adaptation, a dance of resilience, and a tapestry of love.

With a heart full of determination and a spirit full of grace, let us navigate the terrain of returning to work and balancing career and motherhood a terrain that reflects the beauty of balance and the art of embracing change.

Chapter 21:

Sibling Bonding and Family Dynamics

Preparing Siblings for the New Arrival. Fostering a Strong Sibling Relationship.

In the intricate tapestry of family life, the introduction of a new sibling brings forth a chapter of transformation a chapter that unveils the art of preparing existing siblings for the arrival of a new family member and nurturing the bonds that will shape their shared journey. The path of sibling bonding and family dynamics is one of growth, adaptation, and the profound importance of fostering connections that withstand the tests of time. As you embrace the role of parent to multiple children, you embark on a journey that requires intention, understanding, and the ability to navigate the dynamics of a growing family with grace. The journey of sibling bonding and family dynamics is a tapestry that weaves together the threads of preparation, communication, and the celebration of each child's unique presence. Welcome to the realm of sibling bonding a journey that explores strategies for preparing existing siblings for the new arrival and offers insights into fostering a strong and loving sibling relationship.

Preparing Siblings for the New Arrival

The anticipation of a new sibling's arrival is a time of both excitement and adjustment for existing siblings. Navigating this transition with sensitivity and intention can set the foundation for a positive and loving sibling relationship.

Early Communication

- **Timing**: Start discussing the upcoming arrival with your existing children early in the pregnancy. This gives them time to process the news and ask questions.

- **Honesty**: Be honest about the changes that will occur, including the adjustments in routines and the need to share attention.

Involvement and Inclusion

- **Inclusive Language**: Use inclusive language that emphasizes the new baby as an addition to the family rather than a replacement.

- **Involvement**: Involve existing siblings in baby-related activities, such as choosing names, decorating the nursery, or helping with baby gear.

Emotional Preparation

- **Acknowledging Feelings**: Validate any feelings of excitement, apprehension, or jealousy that existing siblings may experience. Let them know that all emotions are valid.

- **Books and Stories**: Read books or tell stories about becoming an older sibling. This helps children understand that their feelings are shared by many.

Fostering a Strong Sibling Relationship

As the new sibling arrives and settles into the family, the journey of fostering a strong sibling relationship begins. Nurturing this bond requires patience, guidance, and the ability to navigate the challenges that may arise.

Sharing Attention

- **Individual Time:** Dedicate individual time to each child. This reinforces that they are loved and valued individually.

- **Sibling Bonding Time**: Encourage sibling bonding time by engaging in activities that they can enjoy together.

Conflict Resolution

- **Teaching Conflict Resolution**: Teach your children healthy ways to resolve conflicts and communicate their feelings.

- **Modeling Behavior**: Model respectful communication and problem-solving for your children to emulate.

Encouraging Mutual Support

- **Teamwork**: Encourage your children to support and help each other. This may include assisting with tasks, sharing toys, or comforting each other.

- **Celebrating Milestones**: Celebrate each child's milestones and achievements to emphasize the uniqueness of their individual journeys.

The Dance of Sibling Connections

As you navigate the intricate terrain of sibling bonding and family dynamics, remember that the journey is an opportunity to nurture connections, instill values, and foster a sense of unity within your growing family.

Nurturing Individuality

While nurturing sibling bonds, it's equally important to honor each child's individuality. Encourage their unique interests, strengths, and aspirations.

Celebrating Togetherness

Celebrate the moments of joy, laughter, and shared experiences as your children embark on the remarkable journey of growing up together.

The Journey of Sibling Bonding Continues

As you navigate the realm of sibling bonding and family dynamics, remember that the path you tread is a reflection of your dedication to nurturing connections, fostering understanding, and celebrating the richness of a growing family.

In the chapters that precede and follow, we have explored the multifaceted landscape of parenting, delving into the art of nurturing your well-being, fostering connections, and embracing the remarkable journey of raising a child. We have unveiled the practices that support you as parents, offered guidance for parenting challenges, and provided insights into the extraordinary journey of parenthood.

As you continue on this remarkable journey, may your children's bonds flourish, may your family thrive, and may your heart be open to the exquisite dance of sibling relationships. Your journey is a symphony of unity, a dance of connection, and a tapestry of love.

With a heart full of unity and a spirit full of grace, let us navigate the terrain of sibling bonding and family dynamics a terrain that reflects the beauty of connection and the art of embracing growth.

Chapter 22:

Beyond Baby Blues: Recognizing Postpartum Depression

Identifying Signs of Postpartum Depression. Seeking Support and Treatment.

In the tapestry of motherhood, the journey of postpartum emotions weaves a complex landscape of highs and lows. Amid the wonder and joy, there are moments of vulnerability and adjustment that are part of the fabric of early parenthood. Yet, for some, the emotional tapestry becomes tangled in the threads of postpartum depression a condition that calls for understanding, support, and the awareness of the profound impact it can have on a mother's well-being. The path of recognizing postpartum depression is one that requires compassion, education, and the ability to identify the signs that distinguish it from the common "baby blues." As you navigate this sensitive terrain, remember that seeking help is an act of courage one that honors your mental health and the sanctity of your journey. Welcome to the realm of recognizing postpartum depression a journey that explores the signs of this condition and offers insights into seeking support and treatment for a brighter path forward.

Identifying Signs of Postpartum Depression

Postpartum depression is a distinct and serious condition that affects a significant number of new mothers. It's important to differentiate it from the common "baby blues," which typically involves mild mood swings and emotional sensitivity. Identifying the signs of postpartum depression is crucial for seeking timely support and intervention.

Emotional Symptoms

- **Persistent Sadness:** Feeling overwhelmingly sad or tearful most of the day, nearly every day.

- **Hopelessness**: A sense of hopelessness or worthlessness that extends beyond the typical challenges of new parenthood.

- **Emotional Numbness**: Feeling emotionally detached from your baby or other loved ones.

- **Intense Irritability:** Experiencing anger, frustration, or irritability that is beyond your usual emotional range.

Physical Symptoms

- **Extreme Fatigue**: Overwhelming exhaustion that persists even with adequate rest.

- **Appetite Changes**: Significant changes in appetite, whether it's a decrease or an increase.

- **Sleep Disturbances**: Trouble sleeping, even when you have the opportunity.

Cognitive Symptoms

- **Difficulty Concentrating**: Finding it hard to focus, make decisions, or think clearly.

- **Negative Self-Image**: Developing negative thoughts about yourself, your abilities, or your worth as a parent.

- **Intrusive Thoughts**: Experiencing distressing or intrusive thoughts that are difficult to control.

Seeking Support and Treatment

Recognizing postpartum depression is the first step toward healing. While it may feel daunting, seeking support and treatment is essential for your well-being and the well-being of your family.

Talk About Your Feelings

- **Open Up**: Discuss your feelings with your partner, family members, friends, or a mental health professional.

- **Normalize Seeking Help**: Understand that seeking help is a sign of strength and self-awareness, not weakness.

Support

- **Therapy**: Consider individual or group therapy, such

as cognitive-behavioral therapy, which can be effective in treating postpartum depression.

- **Medication**: In some cases, medication may be recommended by a healthcare professional to help alleviate symptoms.

Self-Care and Coping Strategies

- **Prioritize Self-Care**: Engage in activities that bring you joy, relaxation, and a sense of purpose.

- **Physical Activity:** Regular physical activity can have positive effects on mood and overall well-being.

- **Support Groups**: Joining a support group for mothers with postpartum depression can provide a safe space to share experiences and insights.

The Path to Healing and Resilience

As you navigate the journey of recognizing postpartum depression, remember that seeking support and treatment is a testament to your resilience and commitment to your well-being.

Reaching Out

Reach out for help even if you're unsure. Sharing your experiences with a professional can provide clarity and guidance.

Nurturing Your Well-Being

Nurturing your well-being is a journey that involves seeking help, practicing self-care, and cultivating a sense of self-compassion.

The Journey of Healing Continues

As you navigate the realm of recognizing postpartum depression, remember that the path you tread is one of empowerment a path that honors your mental health, acknowledges your strength, and offers the promise of a brighter future.

In the chapters that precede and follow, we have explored the multifaceted landscape of motherhood, delving into the art of nurturing your well-being, fostering connections, and embracing the remarkable journey of raising a child. We have unveiled the practices that support you as parents, offered guidance for parenting challenges, and provided insights into the extraordinary journey of parenthood.

As you continue on this remarkable journey, may your well-being flourish, may your resilience shine, and may your heart be open to the exquisite dance of healing and growth. Your journey is a symphony of self-discovery, a dance of courage, and a tapestry of love.

With a heart full of compassion and a spirit full of grace, let us navigate the terrain of recognizing postpartum depression a terrain that reflects the beauty of seeking help and the art of embracing hope.

Chapter 23:

Parenting Styles and Philosophies

Exploring Different Parenting Approaches. Finding What Works for Your Family.

In the intricate tapestry of parenting, the landscape is as diverse as the colors of a sunset. Each family brings their unique essence, values, and aspirations to the journey of raising children. This chapter is an exploration of the kaleidoscope of parenting styles and philosophies the myriad ways in which parents approach the art of nurturing and guiding their children. As you navigate the choices that define your parenting journey, remember that the path is a personal one that honors your values, respects your instincts, and embraces the beauty of diversity. Welcome to the realm of parenting styles and philosophies a journey that invites you to explore different approaches and discover what resonates with the heart of your family.

Exploring Different Parenting Approaches

Parenting is not a one-size-fits-all endeavor. It is an intricate dance of adapting, learning, and evolving in response to your child's needs, your values, and your family's dynamics. The array of parenting approaches and philosophies reflects the diverse tapestry of beliefs and practices that shape the experiences of families worldwide.

Authoritative Parenting

- **Balanced Approach**: Authoritative parents offer clear expectations and rules while also being responsive to their child's needs and emotions.

- **Encouraging Independence**: This approach fosters independence by providing guidance and boundaries while allowing room for exploration.

Permissive Parenting

- **Flexibility**: Permissive parents are often lenient and

flexible, allowing their children more autonomy in decision-making.

- **Nurturing Creativity**: This style can nurture creativity and self-expression but may require a balance to ensure structure and consistency.

Authoritarian Parenting

- **Clear Boundaries**: Authoritarian parents set strict rules and boundaries, often expecting obedience without room for negotiation.

- **Potential Challenges**: While this approach can establish discipline, it may also lead to a lack of open communication and autonomy.

Attachment Parenting

- **Emotional Connection**: Attachment parenting focuses on building a strong emotional connection between parent and child through responsiveness and nurturing.

- **Responsive Care**: This approach promotes co-sleeping, babywearing, and immediate response to a child's cues for comfort.

Unschooling and Child-Led Learning

- **Autonomy in Learning**: Unschooling encourages children to explore their interests and learn through experiences rather than traditional classroom methods.

- **Holistic Learning**: This approach promotes a holistic approach to education that aligns with a child's curiosity and natural development.

Finding What Works for Your Family

As you navigate the terrain of parenting styles and philosophies, remember that there is no one "right" way to raise a child. The heart of parenting is finding an approach that resonates with your values, respects your child's individuality, and creates a harmonious family environment.

Honoring Your Values

- **Reflect on Values**: Consider what values you want to instill in your child. Choose an approach that aligns with those values.

Observing Your Child

- **Individual Needs**: Observe your child's temperament, personality, and preferences. This can guide your approach to discipline and guidance.

Adapting and Growing

- **Flexibility**: Be open to adapting your approach as your child grows and as new challenges arise.

Harmony and Consistency

- **Creating Balance**: Strive for balance and consistency in your approach to parenting. Consistency provides a sense of security for your child.

The Dance of Parenting Styles

As you navigate the intricate terrain of parenting styles and philosophies, remember that the journey is an opportunity to embrace your unique family story a story woven with love, respect, and the commitment to nurturing your child's growth.

Respecting Differences

Respect the choices of other parents, even if their approach differs from yours. Every family's journey is as unique as a fingerprint.

Growing Together

As you explore different parenting approaches, remember that your journey is a voyage of growth a journey that mirrors the growth of your child.

*The Journey of Parenting Styles Continues

As you navigate the realm of parenting styles and philosophies, remember that the path you tread is a reflection of your dedication to fostering a loving, respectful, and thriving family.

In the chapters that precede and follow, we have explored the multifaceted landscape of motherhood, delving into the art of nurturing your well-being, fostering connections, and embracing the remarkable journey of raising a child. We have unveiled the practices that support you as parents, offered guidance for parenting challenges, and provided insights into the extraordinary journey of parenthood.

As you continue on this remarkable journey, may your family's tapestry flourish, may your choices be guided by love, and may your heart be open to the exquisite dance of parenting styles and philosophies. Your journey is a symphony of individuality, a dance of discovery, and a tapestry of love.

With a heart full of respect and a spirit full of grace, let us navigate the terrain of parenting styles and philosophies a terrain that reflects the beauty of diversity and the art of embracing authenticity.

Chapter 24:

Childproofing Your Home: Safety First

Creating a Safe Environment for Your Baby. Essential Childproofing Tips.

In the symphony of parenthood, one note resounds above all others safety. As you welcome your precious child into the world, the sanctuary of your home transforms into a space that nurtures, protects, and guides their early years. Childproofing your home is a melody of vigilance and preparation an art that requires an understanding of potential hazards and the dedication to creating an environment that fosters exploration without compromising safety. The path of childproofing is one that safeguards your child's well-being, offers peace of mind, and honors the sanctity of parenthood. Welcome to the realm of childproofing your home a journey that explores the nuances of creating a safe haven for your baby and offers essential childproofing tips that resonate with the heart of every parent.

Creating a Safe Environment for Your Baby

Your home is not just a dwelling; it's a cocoon of love, growth, and memories waiting to be woven. As you transform your living space into a sanctuary for your baby, consider every nook and cranny that might pose a potential risk.

Nursery Safety

- **Crib Safety:** Ensure the crib meets safety standards and doesn't have any loose parts or gaps that could trap your baby.

- **Soft Bedding:** Avoid soft bedding, pillows, and stuffed animals in the crib to reduce the risk of suffocation.

- **Secure Furniture**: Anchor furniture to the wall to prevent tipping, especially tall dressers and bookshelves.

Kitchen and Dining Area

- **Lock Cabinets**: Install childproof locks on cabinets containing cleaning supplies, sharp objects, and potentially harmful items.

- **Safe Cooking**: Keep pot handles turned inward to prevent accidental spills, and use back burners whenever possible.

- **Cord Safety**: Keep appliance cords and tablecloths out of reach to prevent pulling or grabbing.

Living Room and Common Areas

- **Electrical Outlets**: Cover electrical outlets with safety plugs or outlet covers to prevent accidental shocks.

- **Blind Cords**: Use cordless blinds or secure cords out of reach to avoid strangulation hazards.

- **Secure Furniture**: Ensure heavy furniture is secured to the wall to prevent tipping over.

Essential Childproofing Tips

Childproofing is not just about removing hazards; it's about creating an environment that nurtures exploration and supports your child's growing curiosity.

Explore From Your Child's Perspective

- **Get Down Low**: Crawl around your home to see potential hazards from your child's perspective.

- **Small Objects**: Pick up small objects that could be choking hazards, such as coins, buttons, or small toys.

- **Secure Doors and Drawers**: Install childproof locks on doors and drawers to prevent access to dangerous items.

Stair Safety

- **Baby Gates**: Install gates at the top and bottom of stairs to prevent falls.

- **Carpeting**: Ensure stairs have non-slip surfaces, and consider using carpeting or adhesive stair treads.

- **Supervision**: Always supervise your child when they're near stairs, even if you have gates in place.

Bathroom Safety

- **Toilet Locks**: Install toilet locks to prevent drowning hazards.

- **Temperature Control**: Set the water heater to a safe temperature to avoid scalding.

- **Medication and Toiletries**: Keep medications and toiletries out of reach in locked cabinets.

The Dance of Safety and Exploration

As you childproof your home, remember that the journey is a delicate dance a dance that weaves the threads of safety and exploration into a tapestry of love and nurturing.

Stay Updated

As your child grows and develops new skills, reevaluate your childproofing measures to address changing risks.

Creating Balance

Strive for a balance between a safe environment and the freedom for your child to explore and learn.

The Journey of Childproofing Continues

As you navigate the realm of childproofing your home, remember that the path you tread is a reflection of your commitment to your child's well-being, your dedication to parenthood, and your deep love for your family.

In the chapters that precede and follow, we have explored the multifaceted landscape of motherhood, delving into the art of nurturing your well-being, fostering connections, and embracing the remarkable journey of raising a child. We have unveiled the practices that support you as parents, offered guidance for parenting challenges, and provided insights into the extraordinary journey of parenthood.

As you continue on this remarkable journey, may your

home be a haven of safety and love, may your heart be open to the symphony of exploration, and may your family's tapestry be woven with the threads of care and vigilance. Your journey is a symphony of protection, a dance of anticipation, and a tapestry of love.

With a heart full of watchfulness and a spirit full of grace, let us navigate the terrain of childproofing your home a terrain that reflects the beauty of safeguarding and the art of embracing preparation.

Chapter 25:

Milestone Moments: Baby's Firsts

Celebrating Baby's Developmental Milestones. Documenting and Preserving Memories.

In the symphony of parenthood, each note is a milestone a melody of growth, discovery, and wonder that marks the path of your baby's journey. The first smile, the tentative steps, the first words they are the threads that weave the tapestry of your child's development, and they are the treasures that adorn your heart with the brilliance of parenthood. Milestone moments are not just events; they are the essence of your child's unique story a story that unfolds with every new experience, every tiny triumph, and every leap of growth. The journey of celebrating baby's firsts is an art that transcends time, an embrace that honors the fleeting beauty of childhood, and a legacy that reverberates through the generations. Welcome to the realm of milestone moments a journey that explores the joy of celebrating developmental milestones and the art of documenting and preserving these cherished memories.

Celebrating Baby's Developmental Milestones

From the moment your baby is born, every heartbeat becomes a milestone a moment that beckons celebration and gratitude. As your baby embarks on the remarkable journey of growth and discovery, take delight in commemorating the milestones that illuminate their path.

The Magic of Firsts

- **First Smile**: A smile that melts your heart, a symbol of connection and recognition.

- **First Laugh**: A symphony of joy that resonates with the pure innocence of childhood.

- **First Steps**: The tentative steps that mark the beginning of a journey toward independence.

Language and Communication

- **First Words**: The moment when babbling transforms into the first recognizable word.

- **Communication Milestones**: Celebrate gestures, coos, and interactions that signify growing communication skills.

Motor Skills and Exploration

- **Reaching and Grasping**: The journey of discovering hands and fingers, reaching out to the world.

- **Crawling and Walking**: Commemorate the milestones of mobility, the journey from crawling to those first wobbly steps.

Feeding and Eating Milestones

- **First Taste**: Celebrate the introduction of solid foods, the adventurous exploration of new flavors.

- **Self-Feeding**: Embrace the journey of self-feeding, a step toward independence and self-sufficiency.

Documenting and Preserving Memories

As time dances forward, the magic of baby's firsts unfolds with grace and swiftness. To capture and preserve these precious moments is to create a tapestry of memories that you and your child will treasure for a lifetime.

Photography and Videography

- **Capture Candid Moments**: Embrace the beauty of spontaneous, candid shots that reflect the authenticity of the moment.

- **Create a Photo Diary**: Document each milestone with a dedicated photo diary, tracing the journey from infancy to childhood.

Journaling and Scrapbooking

- **Write Heartfelt Notes**: Record your thoughts, feelings, and reflections about each milestone in a dedicated journal.

- **Create Keepsake Albums**: Craft a scrapbook or digital

album that beautifully showcases each milestone with photos and anecdotes.

Time Capsules and Mementos

- **Create Time Capsules**: Fill a time capsule with mementos and notes to be opened at a future milestone, creating a bridge between past and present.

- **Collect Memorabilia**: Keep souvenirs from each milestone a baby's first outfit, a lock of hair to create a tangible connection to the past.

The Dance of Celebration and Memory

As you celebrate baby's developmental milestones, remember that the journey is a dance a dance that intertwines the present with the future, the fleeting moments with the enduring memories.

Honoring Individuality

Celebrate each milestone as a unique reflection of your child's personality and growth, honoring the beautiful journey of their development.

Involve Loved Ones

Invite family and friends to share in the joy of milestone celebrations, creating a network of support and love around your child.

The Journey of Celebrating Baby's Firsts Continues

As you navigate the realm of milestone moments, remember that the path you tread is one of reverence a path that celebrates the magic of childhood, preserves the echoes of joy, and enriches the legacy you pass down.

In the chapters that precede and follow, we have explored the multifaceted landscape of motherhood, delving into the art of nurturing your well-being, fostering connections, and embracing the remarkable journey of raising a child. We have unveiled the practices that support you as parents, offered guidance for parenting challenges, and provided insights into the extraordinary journey of parenthood.

As you continue on this remarkable journey, may your heart be filled with the music of celebration, may your memories be adorned with the brilliance of milestones, and may your family's tapestry be woven with the threads of love and cherished experiences. Your journey is a symphony of celebration, a dance of joy, and a tapestry of love.

With a heart full of celebration and a spirit full of grace, let us navigate the terrain of milestone moments a terrain that reflects the beauty of growth and the art of embracing memories.

Chapter 26:

Redefining Self-Care as a New Mom

Prioritizing Self-Care Amidst Motherhood. Finding Joy and Fulfillment in Everyday Moments.

In the symphony of motherhood, your role is a growing up an harmonious blend of nurturing, giving, and embracing the boundless love that accompanies the journey. As a new mom, your days are woven with the melodies of caring for your little one, but amidst these harmonies lies an essential note self-care. In the rhythm of caring for your child, it's easy to neglect your own well-being, yet the truth remains: nurturing yourself is not just a gift to yourself, but a testament to the love you pour into your family. Redefining self-care as a new mom is a melody of balance, a dance that honors your needs and celebrates the joy and fulfillment that come with taking care of yourself. Welcome to the realm of redefining self-care a journey that explores the art of prioritizing self-care amidst motherhood and discovering the beauty of finding joy and fulfillment in everyday moments.

Prioritizing Self-Care Amidst Motherhood

As a new mom, self-care is not a luxury; it's a necessity. Prioritizing your well-being is not an act of selfishness; it's an act of love for yourself and for your family.

Reframing Self-Care

- **From Selfishness to Necessity**: Shift the perspective that self-care is selfish. Recognize that caring for yourself enables you to care for your child with more love and presence.

- **Creating Boundaries**: Establish clear boundaries that carve out time for self-care, whether it's a few moments alone or a dedicated activity.

Nurturing Your Physical Well-being

- **Sleep**: Prioritize sleep whenever possible. Rest is a vital component of physical and mental well-being.

- **Nutrition**: Nourish your body with nutritious meals and stay hydrated to sustain your energy levels.

- **Exercise**: Engage in gentle exercises that align with

your postpartum recovery. Activities like walking or yoga can provide rejuvenation.

Finding Joy and Fulfillment in Everyday Moments

Motherhood is not just about tasks; it's about savoring the moments that make up your journey. Finding joy and fulfillment in these moments is a practice that enriches your experience.

Embracing Present-Moment Awareness

- **Mindful Moments**: Practice mindfulness in everyday activities whether it's feeding your baby, enjoying a cup of tea, or taking a walk.

- **Finding Beauty**: Notice the beauty in small things the sunlight streaming through the window, the sound of your baby's laughter.

Cultivating Fulfillment

- **Pursue Passions**: Carve out time for activities you're passionate about, whether it's reading, crafting, or gardening.

- **Friendships and Connections**: Nurture friendships and connect with other moms who understand the journey.

The Dance of Self-Care and Motherhood

As you redefine self-care as a new mom, remember that the journey is a dance that weaves your needs into the fabric of caring for your child, a dance that enriches your experience and enhances your ability to give.

Role Modeling

By prioritizing self-care, you role model to your child the importance of nurturing oneself and others.

Balance as a Compass

Strive for balance, letting your well-being serve as a compass that guides your journey.

The Journey of Redefining Self-Care Continues

As you navigate the realm of redefining self-care, remember that the path you tread is one of empowerment a path that honors your needs, celebrates your growth, and enriches the legacy you pass down.

In the chapters that precede and follow, we have explored the multifaceted landscape of motherhood, delving into the art of nurturing your well-being, fostering connections, and embracing the remarkable journey of raising a child. We have unveiled the practices that support you as parents, offered guidance for parenting challenges, and provided insights into the extraordinary journey of parenthood.

As you continue on this remarkable journey, may your self-care be a melody of love, may your moments be adorned with joy, and may your family's tapestry be woven with the threads of fulfillment and self-compassion. Your journey is a symphony of self-love, a dance of balance, and a tapestry of love.

With a heart full of nurturing and a spirit full of grace, let us navigate the terrain of redefining self-care a terrain that reflects the beauty of well-being and the art of embracing the fullness of your role as a new mom.

Chapter 27:

Cultivating a Lifelong Love of Learning

Nurturing Intellectual Curiosity in Your Child. Early Learning Activities and Games.

In the symphony of parenthood, you hold the conductor's baton, guiding your child through the harmonies of growth, discovery, and learning. As your child's first teacher, you have the privilege of shaping their perspective of the world, igniting their curiosity, and fostering a lifelong love of learning. The journey of nurturing intellectual curiosity is a symphony of exploration a dance that celebrates every question, embraces every discovery, and lays the foundation for a future filled with wonder. Welcome to the realm of cultivating a lifelong love of learning journey that explores the art of nurturing intellectual curiosity in your child and offers a tapestry of early learning activities and games that resonate with the spirit of discovery.

Nurturing Intellectual Curiosity in Your Child

Intellectual curiosity is the spark that ignites the flame of learning. Nurturing this curiosity is not just about providing answers; it's about fostering an environment that encourages questions, exploration, and a genuine thirst for knowledge.

Creating a Curiosity-Friendly Environment

- **Encourage Questions**: Embrace your child's questions with enthusiasm, creating a safe space for them to explore their curiosity.

- **Model Curiosity**: Demonstrate your own curiosity by asking questions, exploring new topics, and sharing your interests.

Cultivating a Growth Mindset

- **Embrace Challenges**: Teach your child that challenges are opportunities for growth, helping them develop resilience and perseverance.

- **Value Effort**: Celebrate effort and progress rather than just focusing on outcomes.

Early Learning Activities and Games

Early learning is a treasure trove of discovery a canvas upon which your child paints their first strokes of knowledge. Engaging in interactive activities and games not only makes learning enjoyable but also lays the foundation for cognitive development.

Sensory Exploration

- **Sensory Play**: Offer a variety of textures, colors, and materials for sensory exploration. From water play to finger painting, sensory activities stimulate cognitive development.

- **Nature Walks**: Take nature walks to explore textures, colors, and the wonders of the natural world.

Language and Communication

- **Read Aloud**: Introduce your child to the world of words by reading aloud together. Let them see the magic of stories and the power of language.

- **Storytelling**: Encourage your child to create their own stories, nurturing their imagination and language skills.

Math and Problem-Solving

- **Counting Games**: Engage in counting games using toys, objects, or even fingers.

- **Puzzles and Blocks**: Introduce puzzles and building blocks to enhance spatial reasoning and problem-solving skills.

Exploration and Science

- **Science Experiments**: Conduct simple science experiments that spark curiosity and encourage observation.

- **Nature Observations**: Explore the outdoors and

observe plants, animals, and insects in their natural habitats.

The Dance of Curiosity and Exploration

As you cultivate a lifelong love of learning, remember that the journey is a dance that celebrates questions as much as answers, a dance that nurtures the spirit of exploration and lays the foundation for a lifetime of curiosity.

Creating Connections

Connect learning to real-life experiences, showing your child how knowledge is woven into everyday moments.

Fostering Independence

Allow your child to explore topics of interest, letting their curiosity guide the learning journey.

The Journey of Cultivating a Lifelong Love of Learning Continues

As you navigate the realm of nurturing intellectual curiosity, remember that the path you tread is one of empowerment—a path that celebrates the magic of discovery, fosters a passion for learning, and enriches the legacy you pass down.

In the chapters that precede and follow, we have explored the multifaceted landscape of motherhood, delving into the art of nurturing your well-being, fostering connections, and embracing the remarkable journey of raising a child. We have unveiled the practices that support you as parents, offered guidance for parenting challenges, and provided insights into the extraordinary journey of parenthood.

As you continue on this remarkable journey, may your home be filled with the joy of exploration, may your child's curiosity be nurtured with care, and may your family's tapestry be woven with the threads of wonder and a lifelong love of learning. Your journey is a symphony of curiosity, a dance of exploration, and a tapestry of love.

With a heart full of curiosity and a spirit full of grace, let us navigate the terrain of cultivating a lifelong love of learning a terrain that reflects the beauty of intellectual growth and the art of embracing the spirit of discovery.

Chapter 28:

Healthy Habits for the Whole Family

Instilling Healthy Eating and Lifestyle Habits. Exercising Together and Staying Active.

In the symphony of family life, health and well-being compose the heartwarming melody that resonates through generations. As a family, you have the remarkable opportunity to craft a legacy of vitality, nurturing habits that empower both your present and future selves. The journey of cultivating healthy habits is a dance a harmonious fusion of nourishing choices, active living, and the shared commitment to a life of well-being. Welcome to the realm of healthy habits for the whole family a journey that explores the art of instilling healthy eating and lifestyle habits, and invites you to embrace the joy of exercising together and staying active.

Instilling Healthy Eating and Lifestyle Habits

The nourishment you provide your family is not just a meal it's an investment in their well-being. Instilling healthy eating and lifestyle habits sets the foundation for a life marked by energy, vitality, and a deeper connection to the rhythms of nature.

Nurturing Nutritional Awareness

- **Balanced Meals**: Embrace the power of balanced meals, rich in fruits, vegetables, lean proteins, and whole grains.

- **Mindful Eating**: Teach your family the practice of mindful eating, savoring each bite and being present at the table.

Exploring Whole Foods

- **Farm-to-Table**: Connect with local farmers' markets to source fresh, seasonal produce that nurtures your family's health and supports your community.

- **Cooking Together**: Engage your children in the process of cooking, fostering a love for whole foods and culinary creativity.

Exercising Together and Staying Active

The dance of active living weaves through the fabric of family life, creating a tapestry of shared experiences and vibrant health. Exercising together not only cultivates strong bodies but also nurtures strong bonds.

Creating Active Traditions

- **Nature Walks**: Embark on family nature walks, exploring trails, parks, and natural beauty.

- **Outdoor Games**: Rediscover the joy of classic outdoor games tag, hide-and-seek, or a friendly game of soccer.

Involve Every Member

- **Fitness Challenges**: Create family fitness challenges that encourage friendly competition and shared achievement.

- **Dance Parties**: Have spontaneous dance parties at home, celebrating movement and joy.

The Dance of Health and Togetherness

As you cultivate healthy habits for the whole family, remember that the journey is a dance that celebrates nourishment and vitality, a dance that intertwines well-being and togetherness in a beautiful symphony.

Shared Commitment

By embracing healthy habits as a family, you cultivate a sense of shared responsibility for well-being.

Connection Through Movement

Exercising together creates opportunities for bonding,

fostering open communication and connection.

The Journey of Cultivating Healthy Habits Continues

As you navigate the realm of healthy habits, remember that the path you tread is one of empowerment a path that celebrates nourishment, embraces movement, and enriches the legacy you pass down.

In the chapters that precede and follow, we have explored the multifaceted landscape of family life, delving into the art of nurturing connections, fostering lifelong learning, and embracing the remarkable journey of parenthood. We have unveiled the practices that support your family's well-being, offered guidance for parenting challenges, and provided insights into the extraordinary journey of nurturing bonds.

As you continue on this remarkable journey, may your family's days be filled with the nourishment of healthy choices, the joy of movement, and the vibrant energy that accompanies a life well-lived. Your journey is a symphony of well-being, a dance of vitality, and a tapestry of love.

With a heart full of nourishment and a spirit full of grace, let us navigate the terrain of healthy habits for the whole family a terrain that reflects the beauty of well-being and the art of embracing health and togetherness.

Chapter 29:

Maintaining Strong Relationships Outside Parenthood

Nurturing Friendships and Social Connections. Rekindling Hobbies and Personal Interests.

In the symphony of parenthood, your role as a parent harmonizes with the many other facets that make up your identity a friend, a partner, an individual with unique passions. Amidst the melodies of raising a child, it's essential to preserve the notes that compose the symphony of your individuality. The journey of maintaining strong relationships outside parenthood is a dance a graceful fusion of nurturing connections, rekindling passions, and weaving the tapestry of your life with the threads of meaningful interactions. Welcome to the realm of maintaining strong relationships outside parenthood a journey that explores the art of nurturing friendships and social connections, and invites you to reignite your hobbies and personal interests.

Nurturing Friendships and Social Connections

As parenthood takes center stage, it's important to remember that the stage is large enough to accommodate the entire orchestra of relationships that define your life. Nurturing friendships and maintaining social connections enriches your experience and provides a valuable support network.

Cultivating Meaningful Connections

- **Prioritize Social Time**: Set aside time for social interactions, whether it's a coffee date with a friend or a virtual catch-up.

- **Stay Connected**: Utilize technology to stay connected, especially with long-distance friends and loved ones.

Quality Over Quantity

- **Nurture Close Bonds**: Focus on nurturing a few close friendships rather than spreading yourself too thin.

- **Mutual Support**: Lean on your friends for support and offer the same in return. Share the journey of parenthood together.

Rekindling Hobbies and Personal Interests

Parenthood doesn't necessitate the abandonment of the hobbies and passions that define you. In fact, integrating these into your life can provide a sense of fulfillment and balance.

Discovering Your Passions

- **Reflect on Interests**: Take time to reflect on the hobbies and activities that once brought you joy.

- **Slow Start**: Begin by dedicating small pockets of time to engage in your hobbies.

Involve Your Family

- **Family-Inclusive Activities**: Explore hobbies that can involve your family. For instance, if you enjoy painting, set up a family art corner.

- **Sharing Passions**: Share stories of your passions with your child, nurturing their curiosity and interests.

The Dance of Relationships and Self-Discovery

As you maintain strong relationships outside parenthood, remember that the journey is a dance that harmonizes the notes of your individuality with the chords of parenthood, a dance that celebrates both your connections and your personal growth.

Balancing Roles

Recognize that being a parent is just one facet of your identity, and nurturing other relationships is equally important.

Fulfillment Through Diversity

Engaging in diverse activities and nurturing various relationships brings a sense of fulfillment and well-roundedness to your life.

The Journey of Maintaining Relationships Outside Parenthood Continues

As you navigate the realm of maintaining

relationships, remember that the path you tread is one of empowerment a path that celebrates connections, embraces personal interests, and enriches the legacy you pass down.

In the chapters that precede and follow, we have explored the multifaceted landscape of family life, delving into the art of nurturing connections, fostering lifelong learning, and embracing the remarkable journey of parenthood. We have unveiled the practices that support your family's well-being, offered guidance for parenting challenges, and provided insights into the extraordinary journey of nurturing bonds.

As you continue on this remarkable journey, may your life's symphony be composed of meaningful relationships, the joy of shared interests, and the vibrant energy that accompanies a life well-lived. Your journey is a dance of connections, a melody of personal growth, and a tapestry of love.

With a heart full of connections and a spirit full of grace, let us navigate the terrain of maintaining strong relationships outside parenthood a terrain that reflects the beauty of meaningful connections and the art of embracing relationships and personal passions.

Chapter 30:

Embracing the Journey: Reflections on Motherhood

Lessons Learned and Wisdom Gained. Celebrating the Incredible Journey of Motherhood.

In the symphony of life, the chapter of motherhood is a composition that weaves threads of love, challenges, growth, and immeasurable joy. As the curtains draw close on this journey, it's time to reflect upon the tapestry you've woven one that tells a story of transformation, resilience, and the unbreakable bond between a mother and her child. The journey of embracing motherhood is a dance a graceful reflection that echoes the lessons learned, the wisdom gained, and the profound celebration of the incredible journey you've undertaken. Welcome to the realm of embracing the journey: reflections on motherhood a journey that delves into the art of embracing the lessons learned, celebrating the remarkable path you've walked, and inviting you to savor the tapestry of love you've crafted.

Lessons Learned and Wisdom Gained

Every twist and turn along the journey of motherhood

has bestowed upon you a treasure trove of lessons. Each challenge, every triumph, and the intricate interplay of both have enriched your perspective and imbued you with a depth of wisdom that only this journey can offer.

Embracing Imperfection

- **The Art of Adaptation**: Motherhood is a masterclass in adapting to the unexpected. Embrace the art of flexibility and celebrate your ability to navigate uncharted waters.

- **Perfection in Imperfection**: Understand that perfection lies not in flawlessness, but in the love and effort you pour into every moment.

Prioritizing Self-Care

- **Nurturing Yourself**: Acknowledge that nurturing yourself is not selfish it's an act of love that replenishes your reserves to give more.

- **Balancing Acts**: Find equilibrium between your role

as a mother and the many other roles that define you.

Celebrating the Incredible Journey of Motherhood

The journey of motherhood is a canvas painted with moments that range from laughter to tears, from quiet introspection to exuberant celebration. Each chapter has brought its own colors to the canvas, and every stroke has contributed to the masterpiece that is your life as a mother.

Embracing Every Chapter

- **Emotional Milestones**: Reflect on the emotional milestones you've experienced, from the exhilaration of birth to the poignancy of the first day of school.

- **Growth and Discovery**: Celebrate the growth both your child's and your own that has accompanied each stage.

Savoring Precious Moments

- **Small Moments, Big Impact**: Recognize that the most

profound moments are often hidden in the seemingly ordinary.

- **Creating Memories**: Seize the opportunity to create cherished memories, whether it's baking cookies together, reading bedtime stories, or sharing laughter-filled meals.

The Dance of Reflection and Celebration

As you embrace the journey of motherhood, remember that the journey is a dance that celebrates growth and wisdom, a dance that honors the evolution of both you and your child.

Honoring Your Journey

Acknowledge that every twist, turn, and detour has shaped you into the extraordinary mother you are today.

Rooted in Love

Your journey is an ode to love a love that knows no

bounds and a love that transcends time.

The Journey of Embracing Motherhood Continues

As you conclude this chapter and embark on the next phase of your journey, remember that the path you tread is one of empowerment a path that celebrates your growth, embraces the lessons you've learned, and enriches the legacy you pass down.

In the chapters that have unfolded, we've explored the multifaceted landscape of motherhood, delving into the art of nurturing well-being, fostering connections, and embracing the remarkable journey of raising a child. We've unveiled the practices that support you as a mother, offered guidance for parenting challenges, and provided insights into the extraordinary journey of nurturing bonds.

As you continue on this remarkable journey, may your heart be filled with gratitude for the path you've walked, the wisdom you've gained, and the unbreakable bond that defines you as a mother. Your journey is a symphony of love, a dance of growth, and a tapestry of cherished moments.

With a heart full of gratitude and a spirit full of grace, let us embrace the terrain of reflections on motherhood a terrain that reflects the beauty of growth and the art of celebrating the incredible journey of love.